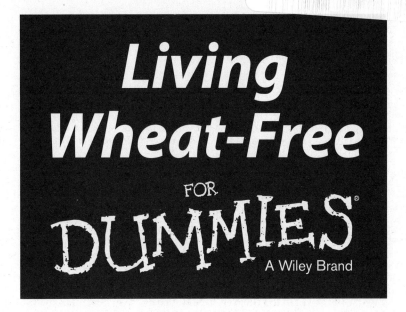

Living Wheat-Free FOR DUMMIES®

A Wiley Brand

by Rusty Gregory, MS, CSCS, CWC
and
Alan Chasen

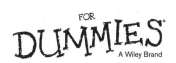

FOR DUMMIES®
A Wiley Brand

Contents at a Glance

Recipes at a Glance

Side Dishes

Appetizers, Snacks, and Dips

Desserts

Table of Contents

Introduction

ntil recently, the healthy-whole-grain mantra has been shouted from the mountaintops with little resistance. Many health "experts" have espoused eating wheat and other grains as a way to achieve good health, gain more energy, and prevent disease.

Now, times are a'changing. With more research comes more insight into the truth behind wheat. Does wheat really provide the nutrition it's believed to? Does it give energy and a better sense of well-being? These questions and so many more are being asked now more than ever. Wheat has officially been put on trial for not living up to its promises of good health, as well as for causing harm to many who consume it.

Sugar and vegetable/seed oils are two other major players in the health decline. Wheat, sugar, and oils together produce a formidable trio that can strip people of their health. In this book, we present the case against all three of these dietary demons and provide you with the information you need to regain control of your health.

The great thing about the changes we hope you're about to embark on is that they have no downside. Only positive effects will take place when you eliminate wheat, added sugar, and vegetable oils. And to those who question your new lifestyle — "But how will you get nutrients and fiber?" — well, we've got you covered there, too.

About This Book

Eliminating wheat and added sugar from your diet may seem like a daunting task at first, but if you're willing, you can do it. The fact that you're reading this book tells us so. The principles we recommend are scientifically sound and presented in a user-friendly way so you can help trump the incorrect conventional wisdom that plagues today's culture.

We provide you with the tools necessary to move from wheat-filled, high-carb eating to wheat-free (and consequently low-carb) eating. We tell you what foods you can eat, what foods to avoid, and why to go cold turkey when removing wheat and sugar from your diet. To help you get started, we include delicious recipes for you and the entire family that are sure to satisfy.

The focus of the book is eliminating wheat from your diet, and that will have an impact on your overall health. To that end, we explain medical tests you may want to discuss with your doctor and what the different results mean. In some places, the material gets a little technical, and we try to make the information as easy to understand as possible. We also offer suggestions for incorporating fitness into your new lifestyle and ways to stick to your wheat-free diet when eating out or sharing meals with family and friends.

We've included information that's interesting but not essential to your new diet in shaded boxes called sidebars. Feel free to skip those. Just because our passion is diet and exercise doesn't mean you have the same depth of interest.

We also use a few conventions in the recipes:

- ✔ All temperatures are Fahrenheit. To convert a temperature to Celsius, type "temperature conversion" into Google. A box will appear at the top of the screen; simply type the Fahrenheit number into the box labeled "Fahrenheit" and the Celsius equivalent will be displayed.

- ✔ When a recipe calls for lemon juice, freshly squeezed juice is the ideal option, but using bottled juice is fine if you're in a pinch.

- ✔ All pepper is freshly ground black pepper unless otherwise noted.

- ☼ Recipes flagged with this icon are vegetarian.

Foolish Assumptions

While writing this book, we made the following assumptions about you and why you're attracted to this topic:

- ✔ You see conflicting information on wheat (and grains in general) and fat in the media and need some clarity.

- ✔ You see food as an important tool to improving your health.

- ✔ The thought of getting the "diseases of aging" — dementia and Alzheimer's — frightens you.

- ✔ You have very little energy, and your body seems to ache all over.

- ✔ You've been applying conventional wisdom to your lifestyle but aren't reaching your health and weight loss goals.

Icons Used in This Book

As you read through the chapters, you see icons — small images in the margins — that are designed to call your attention to specific pieces of information. Here are the icons we use and the kind of information they point out:

This icon marks handy information that will help you avoid wheat or do something better.

This icon calls attention to important details that can make a big difference in following a wheat-free lifestyle.

When you see this icon, we're alerting you to potential problems and common pitfalls of following a wheat-free lifestyle, or to the dangers of not following one.

The information marked with this icon is interesting but not essential to know. If you're the type of person who likes to know everything about everything, you'll enjoy these tidbits. If you want to get the information you need and move on, go ahead and skip these paragraphs.

Beyond the Book

In addition to the material in the print or e-book you're reading right now, this product also comes with some access-anywhere goodies on the web. When you want some quick pointers about living wheat-free, check out the free Cheat Sheet at www.dummies.com/cheatsheet/livingwheatfree. There you'll find lists of restaurants that offer wheat-free meals and lists of other names for wheat and sugar that are used on ingredients labels.

You can find additional information about living wheat-free in some articles that supplement this book. Head to www.dummies.com/extras/livingwheatfree for more information about the steps of the change process, a list of food substitutions to try on your new diet, advice about ordering a wheat-free meal from room service when you're traveling, and a list of ten foods that are billed as healthy but really aren't so good for you.

Where to Go from Here

We've written this book in such a way that you can stop and read any chapter that captures your interest. If you're ready to get started eliminating wheat from your diet, head to Chapter 5. If you want to see how good wheat-free meals can be, turn to Part III and pick out a couple of recipes to try. If you're curious about the health benefits of living wheat-free, check out Chapter 4.

We're convinced that the more you discover about grain-free living, the more you will want to know. You'll find everything you need in this book to help you reach your optimum health.

Part I

Getting Started with Living Wheat-Free

getting started with

living

wheat-free

In this part...

✔ Understand why the key to a healthy lifestyle begins with eliminating wheat, other grains, sugar, and vegetable oils from your diet.

✔ Find out how today's wheat differs from the wheat of generations past and why modern dietary guidelines recommend a significant number of daily servings.

✔ Discover how wheat and gluten are related and realize the difference between a wheat allergy and a wheat intolerance.

✔ See how wheat causes leaky gut and the domino effect of ill health that follows. Get an idea of how wheat and sugar affect blood glucose and insulin.

Chapter 1

Breaking Down the Basics of Living Wheat-Free

In This Chapter

▶ Recognizing the origins and problems of a wheat-heavy diet

▶ Examining how wheat-free eating differs from conventional diet wisdom

▶ Making the change and keeping an eye on the results

▶ Getting started now

*I*magine a world where diabetes, cancer, heart disease, dementia, and Alzheimer's are confined to a fairly small segment of the population. In this scenario, you know maybe one distant family member who suffers from or has died from one of these diseases. Being overweight or obese makes a person an outlier — definitely not the norm.

As fictitious as this world may sound, it was real. Those who grew up prior to the 1960s can usually confirm it. Ask someone from that generation whether he knew anyone back in the day who was overweight, and he can probably name one specific individual. That's how uncommon the condition was.

Unfortunately, the generations that grew up from the 1960s through the present day can be considered guinea pigs in a grand high-carbohydrate, low-fat experiment. Through the 1970s, '80s, and '90s, some misguided science and the resulting governmental guidelines recommended increasing consumption of wheat and grains of all kinds. Fat-free foods loaded with sugar became acceptable for a time, and vegetable oils were encouraged to replace animal fat. All in the name of eliminating fat, especially saturated fat.

To see how those recommendations have turned out, all you have to do is look around you. Chronic diseases such as diabetes, cancer, heart disease, dementia, and Alzheimer's are out of control with no end in sight. These diseases are the leading cause of death and disability in the United States.

Currently, 45 percent of the U.S. population has at least one chronic disease, and 26 percent has multiple chronic conditions. Chronic diseases account for over 80 percent of hospital admissions, over 90 percent of all prescriptions filled, and over 75 percent of all physician visits.

Our goal is to help you to take control of your health and your future, regardless of what current conventional wisdom has to say. Eliminating wheat and other grains, sugar, and vegetable oils will give you the foundation needed to reduce your risk for diseases normally associated with "getting older." From there, you can tweak and modify your diet to fit your lifestyle and needs.

Throughout this book, we talk about the detrimental effects of wheat and other grains. Wheat does seem to cause the most sensitivity for most people, for many reasons we cover in other chapters. With that said, we advise eliminating all grains because of the similarity in their structures. Other grains may not have quite the effect that wheat has, but they still can elicit a response that's not conducive to good health.

How Did We Get into This Wheat Mess? A Brief History

Here's a quick quiz for you: what do George Washington, Ancel Keys, and George McGovern have in common? The answer is wheat.

Each of these men left a lasting legacy with regards to growing, eating, and recommending wheat. George Washington actually perfected growing wheat to take advantage of a shortage in Europe. U.S. exports of wheat totaled in the millions as far back as 1860, setting the stage over the next 150 years for the development of denser wheat plants and denser fields of wheat.

Ancel Keys was an American scientist known early in his career for inventing *K-rations,* the prepared boxes of food the military used in World War II. Ultimately, however, he became better known as the man who started the United States on a path to lowfat eating. His highly controversial beliefs in the 1960s and '70s gained traction thanks to his political connections and convinced many to throw out the butter for a tiny bit of margarine and to up carbohydrate intake (including grains).

The last piece of the wheat puzzle involved the government, specifically Senator George McGovern. In 1977, he released "Dietary Goals for the United States," which encouraged a high-carbohydrate diet (grains and sugar) and a decrease in dietary fat. The recommendations have been tweaked since then, but they essentially remain the same. The ramifications for telling an entire country how to eat can be enormous, especially if the recommendations are wrong. The United States has seen a steady decline in the health of its population since McGovern's guidelines as the prevalence of chronic diseases including heart disease, diabetes, dementia, and Alzheimer's has increased. For a fuller history of wheat's rise to domination, flip to Chapter 2.

Surveying the Health Effects of Wheat and Gluten

"Healthy whole grains" are everywhere. Manufacturers are quick to slap that label across the front of a box regardless of what else is in the product in hopes of convincing consumers that that food choice is healthy. But that conclusion couldn't be further from the truth.

Another buzzword: gluten-free. Wheat and gluten currently are in the public eye more than they've ever been before. Science has revealed that they're responsible for maladies ranging from simple annoying allergies to more-severe conditions such as autoimmune diseases. Knowing the difference between wheat and gluten and where your sensitivities lie is critical as you change your diet.

In the following sections, we overview the true health cost of eating wheat and take a quick look at the wheat/gluten issue.

Glimpsing what wheat does to the body

You hear about the nutrients in grains and the all-important fiber content, but if you look closely, you can see these claims are a bit skewed. Milling and processing reduces many of the nutrients, and the plant's own defenses limit your body's ability to access the remaining nutrients. And grains' insoluble fiber speeds things along the intestinal tract, making the absorption of fat-soluble vitamins more challenging. This scenario is especially important in low-fat, high-fiber diets.

Wheat's impact on blood sugar is shockingly huge. Many people think that to become diabetic, a person must overindulge in sweets and be overweight. It's simply not true. The food recommended by health experts has more of an impact on blood sugar than the candy at the checkout line. Sometimes we wonder whether doctors are even aware of wheat's blood glucose impact. If they were, we think there would be more of a pushback against conventional wisdom. Researchers are discovering blood sugar to be a major long term indicator of all sorts of disease. The consequences of chronically elevated blood glucose lead to gut and brain dysfunction.

Eating wheat may lead to a condition known as *leaky gut syndrome* and what can be called leaky brain syndrome. (See Chapter 4.) Both of these situations result from staples in many people's lives. Stress, wheat and grains, refined carbs, processed foods, antibiotics, NSAIDS, and lack of sleep all contribute to foreign items entering the bloodstream through the gut. When the foreign invaders go where they shouldn't, conditions such as asthma, migraines, arthritis, and depression can follow. These same causes lead to unwanted intruders crossing the blood-brain barrier, which can lead to dementia and Alzheimer's. Until recently, science didn't know the mechanism or testing procedures to determine the extent of this kind of invasion. The picture is quickly unfolding and opening up a whole new understanding of inflammation and its role in autoimmune disease.

With a wheat-free lifestyle, you'll be on your way to healing these possible breaches in your system. In addition, one of the many byproducts of these changes is a reduction in risk for metabolic syndrome, a leading indicator of heart disease (as we discuss in Chapter 4).

When you choose to go completely grain-free, you not only improve your health but also realize how poorly you felt when you were eating a grain-filled diet. Yes, going just wheat-free can help relieve any conditions associated with your past diet. But consider the recommendation to eliminate all grains with this analogy: Someone who has an alcohol problem would never be advised to eliminate only hard liquor but to continue drinking beer. This plan of attack doesn't fix the whole problem.

Differentiating between wheat and gluten

Wheat and other grains contain a protein called *gluten,* which contributes flavor and binding qualities to food, household products, and even toys. One important sub-protein of gluten is *gliadin.* Gliadin causes inflammation and is the initiator of leaky gut in the small intestine. Many people have some sort of sensitivity to gluten, whether it's a little bloating after meals or a complete intolerance (celiac disease). Chapter 3 goes into more detail about the relationship between wheat and gluten and the effects on the body.

The only known cure for gluten-related illnesses is eliminating gluten from the diet, which means eliminating wheat. So going gluten-free means you're automatically wheat-free, but you can be wheat-free without giving up all gluten if you choose. In Chapter 7, you can find lists of foods to throw out of your wheat-free kitchen, including some that include wheat hiding behind sneaky aliases.

Heather's testimonial: Cutting out wheat to cope with chronic disease

The idea of giving up something as fundamental as wheat would've never crossed my mind until my doctor recommended it in 2009. After months of feeling sluggish and experiencing muscle pain, joint aches, and a host of other symptoms, my doctor looked at my most recent blood work and said, "I want you to go three months gluten-free." Having followed her advice, I walked into that three-month follow-up appointment feeling noticeably better. Although I still had symptoms, they weren't as severe. I never expected that she'd tell me I had Sjogren's syndrome and give me prescriptions for six different medications.

After the diagnosis, I fell off the gluten-free wagon. I was too focused on trying to remember to take all my pills at all the right times. Like most patients who receive a diagnosis they're unfamiliar with, I spent a lot of time on the Internet, and I came across some recommendations about a completely wheat-free diet, which were further reinforced by a friend. I decided to try again, simply removing all gluten-containing products at first and later most refined carbohydrates, sugars, and processed vegetable oils.

It took about three months before I really started to feel the change. My rheumatologist told me that I was in remission; he was amazed at the progress I was making in such a short time. I finally convinced him to lower my medication dosages; within the span of a year, I was able to go from six medications to two, one of which I take only as-needed. I'm feeling better than I've ever felt; I'm not just surviving with Sjogren's but thriving with it. I never thought I'd see the day where wheat wasn't part of my life, but I can't argue with the way I feel. This has been one of the best decisions I've ever made, and I only wish I'd made it sooner.

Comparing a Wheat-Free Lifestyle to Other Diets

At some point in time, you or someone you know begins the daunting task of losing weight in order to look and feel better, or for better health. For most, this process means restricting calories to the point of starvation. Yes, you guessed it: the dreaded diet. At first, you're highly motivated to lose those unwanted pounds. But as time passes and you continue to deny your hunger, the motivation fades. That's why so many diets are difficult to follow. Your body's energy demands begin to outweigh the amount of calories your diet of choice allows. Your constant hunger challenges your desire to lose weight and your resolve to stick to your diet, so you experience weakness and a slowed metabolism. You lose your self-control, you give in, and it's adios, diet. Often, you end up gaining more weight and become even more unhealthy than you were before you started.

Having a greater understanding of how wheat, sugar, and vegetable oils affect your weight and health is essential in choosing or developing a diet that will make everyone around you envious. Applying that information to your diet gives you the structure needed to stay the course of good health. Head to Chapter 3 for the specifics.

Many philosophies and diets surrounding food contradict the wheat-, sugar-, and vegetable oil-free lifestyle that's necessary to ensure good health. Understanding the truths behind the more controversial dietary information — such as the idea that red meat is unhealthy, that consumption of fat and cholesterol should be minimized, and that you just have to burn off more calories than you take in — can help you gain confidence in your diet. And confidence is what you need when so many incorrect, mixed messages are swirling around you in every direction.

Mainstream diets can be effective in that they provide a structure with their eating plans. That's not to say that all diets suggest eating healthy foods, however. Quite the contrary. As a general rule, diets restrict calories because of a belief that the less you eat, the less you weigh. The first step to eating less for most plans is reducing the amount of fat. Typically, though, the fat is replaced by wheat-filled offerings.

In Chapter 6, we break down several dietary approaches to see how eliminating wheat and other grains, sugar, and vegetable oils fits into each.

Understanding Lasting Change

Putting a plan into action has its challenges, especially when it involves creating new, healthy routines and dropping old, unhealthy ones such as comfort eating. But, no matter how tough it gets, all these obstacles are greatly overshadowed by the change's benefits.

Success at eliminating wheat and sugar from your diet for good and beginning an exercise program that lasts involves more than just a fleeting thought. It requires determination. When you commit to a new behavior, design a wellness vision, set well-written goals, and have an accountability buddy on board, you create an environment that breeds success. Having a sound understanding of the behavior you're changing will move you to action.

Embracing the tools for change

If you're like most people, at some point you've probably started a new healthy behavior with the best of intentions, only to hit one of life's bumps in the road and end up back at square one. Change can be difficult and is seldom comfortable.

So what's the answer to making a change that lasts? By identifying what's most important to you right now and focusing on that motivation, you set yourself up for big-time success. That one thing that's most important to you — whether it's losing weight, looking great for a special occasion, or improving your health — must evoke an emotional response to keep you committed to reaching your vision.

A few tools can really support your change:

✔ **Stages of Change model:** The *Stages of Change model* helps you identify where you are in the change process and provides techniques to assist you in moving toward lasting change. When you see yourself in a particular stage, structuring your goals accordingly becomes much easier. (Chapter 5 gives you the lowdown on the Stages of Change model.)

✔ **SMART goals and a wellness vision:** Most people set goals flippantly, only to see them fade after a short time. When you set SMART goals, you're much more likely to see your goals through to the end. (SMART is an acronym for specific, measurable, action-based, realistic, and timely.) Writing a wellness vision and setting wellness goals is a way of taking action for your health, not allowing life to just happen to you. You become more focused, motivated, and attentive to the things in life that matter most to you. In Chapter 5, we provide a detailed description on how to write a wellness vision and set SMART goals for your wheat-free lifestyle.

✔ **An accountability buddy:** Finding an accountability buddy has an enormous influence on your commitment to your goals. Making a drastic lifestyle change comes with challenges, whether that's feeling like you need a sugar fix or being tempted to fall back into old routines. An accountability buddy — whether it's your spouse, a family member, a friend, or a coworker — looks out for you and holds your feet to the fire when you can't do it on your own.

Exercising your way to the top of the health charts

Have you ever heard the saying "No train, no gain?" Probably not, because we just made it up. But it speaks to the truth that is found in exercise. As an essential piece to the overall health and well-being puzzle, exercise strengthens the heart, lungs, muscles, bones, and joints. In fact, few systems in the body *aren't* enhanced, strengthened, or improved in some way by exercise.

Exercise has the power not only to improve your health but also to enrich your life and increase your well-being. When you exercise, your thinking, mood, energy, and confidence are all affected for the better. Exercise also helps keep the stress hormone (cortisol) at bay, which aids in stress reduction.

As you age, you become more insulin-resistant to the foods you eat. Exercise allows your cells to be more sensitive to insulin, which decreases your chances of becoming insulin-resistant even as you age. This shift reduces your risk of a whole host of diseases, including Type 2 diabetes.

When you're ready to add exercise to your wheat-free lifestyle, refer to Chapter 16. There, you can find everything you need to start and sustain a program that meets your health needs.

Keeping Your Cool in Special Situations

After you gather all the information you need to get started on your wheat- and grain-free adventure, you can apply it to your daily routine. But sometimes situations pop up that challenge your new lifestyle. For example, dining out can make you feel like you've lost control. The following sections introduce some situations where you may have to put a little more thought into eating wheat-free.

Eating away from home

Even though specific challenges arise when you're eating out, keeping your focus on your commitment to good health can help you weather the storm. The evolution of restaurants to meet the needs of patrons with food sensitivities has grown tremendously since 2000. Restaurants are increasingly offering gluten-free menus and are often more receptive to special ordering (at least in mainstream places). However, the cost of providing items such as grass-fed beef, organic chicken and produce, and wild-caught fish is still prohibitive for a lot of restaurants. If all else fails, just shoot for the best possible alternative so you can focus on enjoying gatherings with family and friends.

Know what restaurants and international cuisines suit your wheat-free lifestyle. Doing so prevents you from showing up at a restaurant and being disappointed by the menu. Although they're not known for their contributions to good health, even some fast food restaurants offer gluten-free items on their menu, so do some research.

If you don't know what ingredients are in a dish, ask. By doing your homework before you get to the restaurant, you can better enjoy those you're dining with. But if you don't have the opportunity to check things out ahead of time — maybe the restaurant was a last-minute choice — don't be shy. Speak to the chef and the manager and tell them what your needs are. Chapter 14 spells out specific questions to ask the restaurant staff to ensure a wheat-free experience.

In due time, you're sure to face the challenge of staying wheat-free while traveling, which requires some careful planning on your part. Having a clear understanding of your trip's itinerary will help determine whether you can grocery shop before or while you're on the trip and what kinds of restaurants and hotel food you'll have access to. You can find tips on planning your diet while traveling in Chapter 14.

Developing an eating plan of action for special occasions

Outlasting the holidays or a special occasion on a wheat-free diet can seem like pure drudgery. With all the foods you no longer eat easily within your reach, you must draw upon your new energy and good health to pull you through. Even the most well-intentioned wheat-avoiders face the challenges of how to eat healthfully when special occasions arise. That's why you need to think ahead about how (and how much) you're going to stick to your guns when celebrations come calling.

The pressures to give in and the inconvenience of having an alternate plan can be overwhelming. As we note in Chapter 15, some people can fudge a little during the holidays or a family gathering without going completely off the dietary rails. If that's you, just be sure to keep a tight rein on your minor indulgences so they don't become a full-fledged backslide.

If you prefer to follow a stricter wheat-free plan (or you must because of a condition such as celiac disease), you can help your cause by establishing strategies such as bringing a wheat-free dish or two, eating the healthiest wheat-free foods first, or hosting the celebration yourself.

Take care when alcohol enters the gathering. Overindulging can cloud your thinking and inhibit your decision-making process when it comes to food consumption.

Business dinners and work functions can be just as difficult to remain wheat-free at, whether it's a corporate seminar or an office baby shower. Making your needs known to the person in charge of planning the meal is critical, as we explain in Chapter 15.

When you eliminate wheat and other grains, sugar, and vegetable oils from your diet, you experience weight loss, feel an increase in energy, and see an improvement in your general health. So much so that you'll probably want to tell the whole world about it. But be sensitive to the fact that some people are skeptical or downright unaccepting of the wheat-free lifestyle. In Chapter 15, we give you advice on spreading the word and answering your critics without force-feeding your message.

Monitoring and Enhancing Your Progress

Some effects of a wheat- and sugar-free diet, such as weight loss and a general feeling of well-being, are pretty noticeable. But how do you know whether your blood sugar or cholesterol numbers have improved? The only way to measure these kinds of markers is to have them tested medically. The following sections preview the benefits of testing and consider a couple of supplements that may help further your improvement.

Checking your progress with basic tests

Buying into the science of a wheat- or grain-free diet and implementing the program are the two toughest obstacles to becoming wheat-free. Identifying yourself as someone who chooses not to eat wheat or sugar is part of that process as well. After a few months of your new lifestyle, the results will start rolling in. As you waltz into the doctor's office to hear the positive results of your blood tests, odds are he'll ask you what type of lowfat diet you're on. Watch his surprised reaction when you tell him you're eating a lower-carb, high-fat diet.

The lipid panel is a common medical test, and its results help you see how your health is improving on a wheat- or grain-free diet. This blood test measures overall cholesterol, LDL (low density lipoproteins), HDL (high density lipoproteins), and triglycerides. Conventional wisdom holds that certain numbers should be high, and other numbers should be low (we get into the specifics in Chapter 17). However, you really need to pay attention to two numbers as they relate to each other. Of all the numbers in the basic lipid panel, the triglyceride-to-HDL ratio gives you the most accurate look at your risk of developing heart disease. And how do you get that ratio to desirable levels? With a wheat/grain-free lifestyle.

Other medical tests that can give you a clear view of your overall health include C-reactive protein, fibrinogen, Lp(a), homocysteine, hemoglobin A1C, and iron. Head to Chapter 17 for more about these tests.

Adding some extras to ensure your progress

Despite what many people want to believe, taking a pill of any kind won't solve your problems. The same is true for taking a supplement or vitamin. In no way are these items a substitute for eating a healthy wheat-free, sugar-free diet. However, they may help you achieve your goals in conjunction with your lifestyle change.

The two most important supplements are fish oil and cod liver oil. *Fish oil* is derived from the tissues of oily fish; salmon, sardines, herring, anchovies, and mackerel have some of the highest ratios of omega-3 fatty acids to omega-6 fatty acids. The desirable ratio shouldn't exceed 4:1 (and ideally, 1:1). Most Americans are closer to 20:1 omega-6 to omega-3. This type of ratio leads to inflammation, which in turn leads to myriad diseases. (You can read more about fatty acid ratios in Chapter 18.)

Cod liver oil, on the other hand, is derived from — you guessed it — the liver of cod fish. Cod liver oil doesn't contain as much of the beneficial omega-3 fatty acids as fish oil does, but it has ample amounts of the fat-soluble vitamins A, D, and K2, which contribute to vital body functions.

Going Wheat-Free: A Quick-Start Guide

Throughout the course of this book, we provide detailed information about how and why you want to go wheat-free. To whet your wheat-free appetite, here's an abridged version of how to accomplish your goal right now.

1. **Clean out your kitchen.**

   Your refrigerator, freezer, and pantry must be void of wheat, added sugar, and vegetable oils so you have no temptations to your new way of life. (While you're at it, we suggest chucking out all grain products entirely.) Why risk getting derailed? Check out Chapter 7 for tips on accomplishing this task.

2. **Head to the grocery store to restock the kitchen.**

   Your items are going to come from the perimeter of the store, where the fresh fruits, veggies, meats, and dairy reside. A few essentials we recommend you always have on hand are pasture-raised eggs, coconut oil, grass-fed beef, dark leafy greens, and an assortment of organic berries.

You may also want to buy an assortment of nuts, cheeses, raw veggies, dark chocolate, and Greek yogurt to have on hand for snacks. Your snacking needs go way down from your norm when you're wheat-free, but sometimes it's nice to nosh a little. For a complete list of wheat-free go-tos, refer to Chapter 7; for our top ten, hit Chapter 20.

Before you head to the store, look over the recipes in Chapters 8 through 13 for some menu ideas. Use the ingredient lists to make a shopping list.

3. **Optional: Get the tests listed in Chapter 17, such as a basic lipid panel.**

    Sometimes getting a lipid panel is as easy as walking into your local drugstore. Although it's not necessary, it's a good way to get a baseline for your health markers so you can track your progress.

4. **Start thinking about your exercise plan as outlined in Chapter 16.**

    Make a trip to the nearest gym or head to a fitness equipment store if you plan to work out at home. Exercise is an integral part of your success, so don't delay.

We're basically recommending going back to a low-to-no-grain, low-sugar, high-fat diet that was far more common more than 50 years ago. Just return to the habits that were once prevalent, where real food was the norm and very few people ate anything out of a box or from a drive-through window.

Transitioning to a wheat-free lifestyle isn't easy. We know that. Though we encourage going cold turkey, we know everyone has missteps along the way. It's a process that evolves over time as you get more and more comfortable with what you can and can't eat — or rather, choose to eat and not eat.

Chapter 2

Connecting Modern Wheat to Modern Problems

In This Chapter

▶ Tracing wheat's changes through time

▶ Understanding why the United States eats so much wheat

▶ Considering wheat's ties to some of today's health crises

*B*rowsing the grocery aisles quickly reminds you about one thing: Wheat is everywhere. Venture away from the perimeter of the grocery store, where items like dairy products, meat, and fresh fruits and veggies are stocked, and lo and behold, every label seems to have some form of wheat in it. Currently, only corn consumption exceeds wheat consumption, and that's because corn has other uses such as feeding livestock and making ethanol.

In this chapter, we explain how wheat was around for thousands of years with only modest changes. The last century changed all that with highly processed milling that uses chemicals and additives that pose health risks.

Not Your Grandpa's Wheat: Checking Out Wheat's Evolution

The days of wheat blowing tall in the wind are gone. *Dwarf* and *semi-dwarf* wheat (shorter varieties created to help combat world hunger) comprise more than 99 percent of the wheat worldwide. Wheat that once grew wild can now only grow with human support from pest controls and fertilizers, leaving an inferior product that doesn't resemble what earlier generations ate when they were young. Wheat has changed so much through the years that "the staff of life" is anything but, as we explain in the following sections.

Going back to wheat's roots

Though the modern version of wheat has been around since the early 1960s, history shows that humans have been eating the original wild version going back 10,000 or 11,000 years. In fact, the Middle East (primarily southeast Turkey) can claim early dibs on this crop.

The ancestor of modern wheat was known as *einkorn*. The Natufians, who roamed much of the Middle East, made use of not only einkorn but also wild cereals and rye. The climate in the area allowed them to cultivate the seeds and plan for the long term. Most people at that time were hunters and gatherers, but the Natufians used the wheat as a staple, and it helped them thrive and create the first settlements.

Einkorn gave way to another form of wheat called *emmer*. Emmer was abundant in more varied climates, including cooler weather. It became the dominant wheat in many parts of the Middle and Far East and Europe until about 4000 to 1000 BCE.

Spelt arrived on the scene around the fifth or sixth century BCE; because of its wild grass parents, it had a superior adaptability to its wheat predecessors. Finally, the early wheat varieties concluded with *triticum aestivum,* also known as common bread wheat. Today's wheat is in this form, even though *triticum aestivum* originally appeared about 1700 BCE.

Milling away the nutritional value

Wheat remained relatively the same until the population explosion after the end of the Napoleonic Wars in 1815. In their desire to make chemical fertilizers, European chemists inadvertently poisoned the soil because they didn't understand the science of what they were doing. Through the 19th century, more wars, a potato blight, and a cholera epidemic resulted in food shortages in France and England.

America was in a perfect position to take advantage of Europe's needs. Thanks in part to George Washington, wheat was readily grown and cultivated with superior crop rotations and fertilizers. (*Crop rotation* refers to Washington's seven-year plan to vary the crops planted and keep the soil nutrient dense.) His methods also increased the wheat yield. With new techniques and virgin soil, America was off and running in the export business. By 1860, America was exporting millions of bushels of wheat to many parts of the world.

The increased demand and the advent of the industrial age reduced the cost of production for many foods, whether by speeding up the process or using cheap ingredients. Many times these ingredients were items such as aluminum sulfate or wood shavings that were downright dangerous.

Seeing what's used to process wheat

Many chemicals and other substances are used to mill and process wheat. Here's a list of the most common ones used:

- Ammonium chloride
- Azodicarbonamide
- Benzoyl peroxide
- Calcium propionate
- Chlorine dioxide
- Dextrose
- Diacetyl tartaric acid
- Esters of mono and diglycerides
- Gluten (extra added)
- Potassium bromate
- Sodium stearoyl 2 lactylate
- Starch enzymes

The need for longer lasting flour led grain producers to remove the outer bran and germ layer, which contain most of the nutrients.

The impact of the commercial bakers loomed large because times were changing. In America, for instance, 70 percent of all bread eaten in 1910 was baked at home. By 1924, that figure was 30 percent. By 1930, Wonder Bread came sliced and in a protective wrapper. The highly processed bread was enriched with vitamins and minerals to help fight deficiency conditions, especially those related to B vitamins. Wheat, which had once been a fairly nutritious grain, now required enrichment to achieve the level of quality that existed in the pre-processing era.

Today, wheat is bleached by using questionable ingredients to make better-tasting bread with a longer shelf life and a desirable texture. The end result is a low-nutrient-quality product whose ingredients have serious side effects.

Modifying wheat's genetics to increase yields

The processing involved with wheat is only part of the problem. In an effort to end world hunger in the mid-20th century, finding ways to increase grain yields became a priority. Norman Borlaug, who would eventually win a Nobel Peace Prize for his efforts, began using heavy amounts of nitrogen fertilizer. The resulting wheat stalks were tall with lots of grain on the tops. Unfortunately, they tended to collapse from the excess weight.

To solve the toppling-over problem, dwarf and semi-dwarf wheats were developed through genetic modification. The ability to feed the world was becoming a reality. However, a tradeoff of the new wheat strains is a much lower nutrient density. In fact, these wheats have 20 to 30 percent less nutrient content than traditional wheat. Nutrients such as zinc, iron, magnesium, manganese, sulfur, phosphorous, and calcium are all affected. Scientists have been unable to decrease wheat's levels of phytates, which bind to nutrients and make them indigestible to humans. Nutrients otherwise measured in the grains may not be usable because of the phytates.

The modern dwarf wheat poses one other problem: It also contains much higher amounts of the genes for *gluten,* the protein associated with celiac disease. The hybridization that has taken place to achieve higher yields doesn't seem to be as clean as scientists thought. When wheats are combined, 95 percent of the new genes are from the parents, but the other 5 percent aren't. This unique 5 percent is what can cause the gluten proteins to undergo considerable change.

Analyzing the Consumption Explosion

The differences between the wheat of yesteryear and the wheat used in processed foods today explain the negative effects modern wheat has on the body. To avoid these negative effects, all you have to do is eat less wheat, right? Not so fast. Most of the Western world is consuming more calories and becoming less healthy. Americans are eating an average of 10 percent more calories now than in 1970. Half of those additional calories come from wheat and other grains, but the other half come from sugar.

The rise in wheat and sugar consumption has several explanations: infighting in the scientific community, government nutrition guidelines, and subsidies for particular crops. We cover these in more detail in the following sections.

Escalating the diet wars

The man considered to be most responsible for the changes to the American diet is Ancel Keys, an American scientist. Keys became famous for the invention of *K-rations,* the boxed meals given to World War II soldiers. He turned his attention to diet and heart disease beginning in the late 1940s. By the early 1950s, he was speaking about the connection of fat and cholesterol in the blood to heart disease, even though the medical community was split on this link at the time of his initial findings.

Keys's focus was on his famous Seven Countries Study, which he claimed proved the fat/heart disease link. How Keys came to his conclusions has always spurred a lot of controversy, but even without the consensus of the scientific community, he soon found believers in the politicians of the day.

Keys's archrival in the diet wars was John Yudkin, a British physiologist and scientist. Yudkin spent most of the 1960s researching the effects of sugars and starches on animals and people. His findings culminated with the release of his book *Pure, White and Deadly* in 1972. He asserted that blood sugar levels and *triglycerides* (fat in the blood caused by eating carbohydrates) were more dangerous than the consumption of fat and cholesterol in regard to heart disease. He linked sugar and starches directly to Type 2 diabetes and obesity. By the time Yudkin published his book, his theory was in direct opposition to Keys's theories, which had been accepted by the medical community as fact.

People took sides on the issue, with Europeans tending to side with Yudkin and Americans tending to side with Keys. What many didn't realize was that much of the data used to prove Keys's fat theory simultaneously proved Yudkin's sugar theory.

Guiding to the grain

Enter Senator George McGovern, the chairman of the Senate Select Committee on Nutrition and Human Needs. The committee members were focused on trying to solve malnutrition in the mid-1970s when they found their mission coming to an end. Before the group disbanded, they decided to create some nutritional standards and policy for the United States.

After hearing expert testimony from both sides of the high-fat/low-fat argument, McGovern wanted to come to a consensus that the scientific community couldn't. Rates of obesity and diabetes had taken an upward swing earlier in the decade, and he felt changes needed to be made on a national level before things got worse. McGovern employed a young staff writer with no training in science writing or health and nutrition to finalize some recommendations. The writer consulted Harvard nutritionist Mark Hegsted, who convinced him that low-fat eating was the way to go.

What followed in 1977 was a report entitled "Dietary Goals for the United States." The new recommendations were as follows:

✔ Increase carbohydrate intake to 55 to 60 percent of calories. ("Carbohydrate intake" included grains, fruits, and vegetables.)

✔ Decrease dietary fat intake to no more than 30 percent of calories.

✔ Decrease cholesterol intake to 300 milligrams per day.

✔ Decrease sugar intake to 15 percent of calories.

✔ Decrease salt intake to 3 grams per day.

Meat and dairy producers were obviously upset with the government's report. What had been staples in the American diet were now portrayed as villains to the country's health. The National Academy of Sciences (NAS) Food and Nutrition Board felt, like many nutritionists, that the government shouldn't get involved with what should be a scientific recommendation. They felt that people should be instructed to consult with their physicians on nutritional matters and that evidence didn't exist to recommend reductions in fat and cholesterol.

Soon after, the NAS issued a rebuttal report called "Toward Healthful Diets." The U.S. Department of Agriculture claimed the NAS had ties to the food industry, and public perception favored the new Dietary Goals. The meat and dairy industries got the bad end of the deal, while the grain industry came out on top. In the United States, wheat was now supposed to be the answer.

The Dietary Goals for the United States gave way to the Dietary Guidelines, which would be issued every five years. The grain recommendations before 1977 were four servings per day. By 1984, the guidelines recommended 6 to 11 servings of grains per day, while recommending a total of only 2 to 3 servings of meat, poultry, fish, beans, eggs, and nuts per day. During the 1980s and 1990s, fat was removed from practically everything to appeal to those on a low-fat diet; however, the fat was replaced with sugar and, usually, refined grains to help maintain the flavor lost with the fat.

Alan's journey to living wheat-free

I, Alan, was an overweight child. By today's standards, I would've blended right in with most of the population, but growing up in the 1970s made me more of a physical exception. Being very aware of my weight, I attended Weight Watchers at the tender age of 9. The time frame coincided perfectly with the governmental recommendations outlined in the nearby section "Analyzing the Consumption Explosion."

I followed the guidance to a T. I ate grains and sugar- and fat-free everything. Because I was so intent on losing weight, I ate very, very small portions. My daily calorie levels were so low that I probably could've eaten anything and seen results. The difference was that the grains and sugar were making me want to eat more and more, so daily life was miserable. There was no fat in my diet to satisfy my hunger. Food was all I could think about 24 hours a day. The human body can only keep that up for a short time and, as a determined child, I made it about three weeks. As I grew, I was able to keep my weight at a normal level through limited-calorie diets and exercise, especially weight training.

Throughout my college years and my studies thereafter, the focus was still on lowering fat intake for weight loss.

Not until 2009 did I learn about grain's and sugar's effect on weight. It was like a spiritual awakening. Cutting these from my diet allows me to keep my weight under control with zero effort. Previously, my high-grain/high-carb diet forced me to eat every three to four hours. Now I eat when I'm hungry, about every eight to ten hours. And I never feel ravenous hunger — just mild hunger.

Through it all, I feel lucky that I didn't allow myself to be a victim of self-blame. Most who grew up overweight in the past few generations can't claim that. People thought being overweight stemmed from a lack of willpower; the solution was to exercise more and push away from the table. Not being able to do those two simple things indicated some sort of moral deficiency. The sad truth is that eating the "right" things was what made us overweight. I was a living example.

Subsidizing crops for the good of mankind

During the Great Depression, the U.S. government offered subsidies to farmers to prevent them from going bankrupt. The government paid farmers to not grow crops, causing prices to remain elevated. Since then, agricultural subsidies have morphed into various forms, depending on the perceived needs of the grain growers. These agricultural supports favor mass-produced grains that provide the majority of calories as recommended by governmental guidelines. Unfortunately, these supports don't extend to the organic farmers who grow healthier vegetables, which creates an unequal playing field for those trying to provide the best food possible.

Today, the top three subsidized crops in America are

- **Corn:** Corn output consists mostly of high fructose corn syrup (HFCS), also known as corn sugar. HFCS was once touted as a healthy alternative to sugar, though it now has a much more negative reputation. Corn is also used for livestock feed, even though it's not a natural part of a cow's diet.

- **Wheat:** Subsidies encourage high-yield dwarf wheat to maximize crops.

- **Soybeans:** Most soybeans are used to make soybean oil. Of all the oil consumed in America, 65 percent is from soybeans.

It doesn't take a detective to notice that subsidies favor grains, sugars (through HFCS), and factory-raised (corn-fed) meats. Vegetables, fruits, and nuts are nowhere to be found. Why would farmers plant vegetables and fruits when they know they can get higher subsidies for growing wheat or corn?

However, the consequences of consuming greater amounts of corn, wheat, and soybeans (in the form of partially hydrogenated oil) can't be ignored.

- High fructose corn syrup increases inflammation and blood glucose levels, leading to weight gain and diabetes. Corn-fed livestock is more susceptible to diseases that require antibiotics. The cows' poor nutrition also leads to lower levels of healthy omega-3 fatty acids in the meat.

- Wheat causes blood glucose levels to rise, and inflammation follows. Additionally, the popular high-yield dwarf wheat that boosts yields actually minimizes the wheat's nutrition.

- Soybean oil contains high levels of omega-6 fatty acids, which leads to inflammation.

The mass production of these subsidized crops and their use in processed foods lead to cheaper items on grocery shelves and at fast-food restaurants. So why would a consumer choose grass-fed beef and broccoli when the far cheaper alternative is a combo meal of meat from malnourished cows on a bun made from dwarf wheat with a side of potatoes fried in omega-6-laden oil and a soda containing 100 percent high fructose corn syrup? Sadly, the real answer is that many Americans don't have a choice financially, and subsidies don't favor healthy eating.

More Wheat, More Problems: Linking Wheat to Health Epidemics

All foods are made up of carbohydrates, proteins, and/or fats. Cutting back on one type means making up the difference with the other two. So when the push came in the 1970s to reduce fat intake, carbs or protein had to pick up the slack. Inevitably, carbs — often unhealthy ones in the form of modified wheat — were the next choice. These changes have resulted in significant health declines across the population.

In the following sections, we give you the alarming statistics resulting from the increased consumption of wheat and how it has contributed to the health problems of the U.S. population. We go into more details about wheat's effect on health in Chapter 4.

A growing epidemic: Tackling weight gain and obesity

When people reminisce about growing up in the 1940s or 1950s, they talk about meals consisting of pasture-raised meats; vegetables from the back-yard or local market; and lots of butter, cream, and even lard. They may also mention that the bread at the table had a different texture and taste than today's bread. They don't, however, usually talk about the large numbers of overweight people they saw. That reality just didn't exist.

Today, the experience is different. Many friends and relatives are overweight and maybe even obese. You may be heavier than you and your doctor want you to be (maybe that's why you're reading this book). According to the National Health and Nutrition Examination Survey, 40 percent of men and 28 percent of women were overweight in 2012; in addition, another 34 percent of men and 36 percent of women were obese. As for children, a third of them between the ages of 2 and 19 were overweight, with 18 percent of those being obese. This number represents a fivefold increase since the early 1970s.

Being overweight is defined as having more body fat than is optimally healthy. Being obese is defined as having excess body fat that is likely to lead to reduced life expectancy and increased health problems. The concern is for the overweight individual who is leading an unhealthy lifestyle that furthers the weight gain, leading to obesity.

Obesity itself is a health condition, but it also contributes to other medical woes. The following are modern-day diseases that are affecting more people every day and are closely related to the obesity epidemic:

- Alzheimer's disease
- Arthritis
- Cancer
- Diabetes
- Heart disease
- Hypertension
- Metabolic syndrome (high triglycerides, abdominal fat, high blood pressure, insulin resistance)
- Stroke

Obesity's costs in dollars to the United States are huge. Americans spend about $150 billion annually in health care tied to obesity alone, with an additional $75 billion in lost productivity. Research shows that those who are obese take more sick days and are less effective while at work, which reduces productivity. If trends in obesity continue, these costs will only go up and pose more challenges to an already-stressed health care system.

Obesity: An expanding problem around the globe

On a worldwide scale, the Western diet has become a global diet. Globalization means that fast food full of wheat, sugar, and vegetable oils is sprouting all around the world. Countries such as France and Japan have seen their childhood obesity rates double over four decades. Obesity has actually replaced malnutrition as the number one problem in poorer countries.

Is the entire world turning into one big couch potato? Is everyone on earth losing the ability to exhibit self-control? Or are the foods themselves making people obese?

Seeing the rise of diabetes

The accelerated rates of obesity are causing a rise in the rates of diabetes. Not every person who is obese will get diabetes, but carrying too much weight is a major contributor. Thin Type 2 diabetics exist, but they are far more the exception than the norm.

More than 8 percent of the general U.S. population has diabetes. (When we refer to diabetes, we're referring to Type 2 diabetes; check out Chapter 4 for info on how Type 2 differs from Type 1.) And because diabetes doesn't occur overnight, another 89 million people are on the path to diabetes, also known as prediabetes. The highest rates occur in the oldest populations; in the over-65 age group, the known diabetes rate is 27 percent.

Worldwide, the diabetes rate is 8 percent and growing rapidly. In 2013, nearly 382 million people around the world are diabetic, and that's just the number who've been diagnosed; an estimated 175 million cases of diabetes are undiagnosed. Of those who are diagnosed, 50 percent die before age 60. These statistics are meaningful, and they're preventable.

Your gut run amuck: Diagnosing digestive ailments

Two digestive conditions are made worse by gluten, a protein found in wheat. The first, which most people have heard of, is celiac disease. Celiac is an autoimmune disorder that occurs in genetically predisposed people. When someone with celiac disease is exposed to the gluten protein, enzymes in the body modify the protein to the point of resembling intestinal tissue; inflammation follows. Celiac disease can be diagnosed with medical tests and a biopsy of the intestines.

Celiac disease affects about 1 percent of the population. That's four times the rate from the 1960s. Beyond the 1 percent, estimates say that about six times that number go undiagnosed or misdiagnosed with other conditions. It can take up to 20 years to be properly diagnosed with celiac disease.

The second condition affected by gluten is non-celiac gluten sensitivity (NCGS). Like celiac disease, NCGS is caused by the body's reaction to gluten, but the reaction isn't autoimmune or an allergy. Unlike celiac disease, no diagnostic test is available for NCGS.

NCGS can affect almost every tissue in the body, including the brain, stomach, skin, liver, muscles, and thyroid. It's also associated with a variety of diseases, including epilepsy, Type 1 diabetes, osteoporosis, conditions of the nervous system, thyroid, and schizophrenia.

Because NCGS is fairly new, many doctors don't acknowledge it. For them, it's a cut-and-dried measure: you either test positive for celiac, or you don't; if you don't, gluten isn't a problem for you. The symptoms for celiac disease and NCGS are nearly identical, which complicates diagnosis of NCGS. Symptoms of both diseases include

- ✔ Abdominal cramping and gas
- ✔ Achy joints
- ✔ Depression
- ✔ Diarrhea
- ✔ Fatigue
- ✔ Headaches
- ✔ Weight loss

Doctors and patients don't always make the link between these symptoms and gluten because the symptoms are so diverse and can appear so random. Often, a condition unrelated to gluten is given as the diagnosis without regard to the root cause. However, with so many diseases like diabetes, osteoporosis, and thyroid conditions on the rise since the advent of modern wheat, thinking about how the changes to wheat play a role is only logical. (For details on how wheat has changed for the worse over time, flip to the earlier section "Not Your Grandpa's Wheat: Checking Out Wheat's Evolution.") The only true way to confirm these symptoms as a wheat-related problem is to remove the wheat from your diet (under a doctor's supervision) and monitor how you feel.

Chapter 3

Separating the Wheat from the Gluten

*Y*ou've probably heard a lot about wheat and gluten and their detrimental effects on the human body; these two can pack a powerful punch. Understanding who these two culprits are and where to find them is a vital step in eliminating them from your diet.

In this chapter, we explain how wheat and gluten are different and why those differences are important. We also dig into the purposes of gluten in foods and products. We discuss some of the conditions and diseases associated with wheat and gluten consumption and how to treat them. Finally, we discuss how a wheat- or grain-free diet differs from a gluten-free diet and the foods that need to be avoided and can be included in both.

Recognizing that Wheat and Gluten Aren't the Same

Because they're closely related, the words *wheat* and *gluten* are often used interchangeably to describe sensitivities or allergies to certain foods. But this usage is incorrect and causes a lot of confusion. *Wheat* is a cereal grain and made up of carbohydrates. *Gluten* is a large protein, made up of smaller proteins, that gives food its elasticity.

In the following sections, we explain what gluten is and why it's found in so many foods. Then we explain why you need to understand what the terms *wheat-free, grain-free,* and *gluten-free* mean in terms of your diet.

Of the three, grain-free is the most restrictive.

Defining gluten and its uses

Gluten is a grouping of proteins found in wheat, barley, and rye. Some people are known to be sensitive to certain types of gliadin, one of the proteins that make up gluten. In food preparation, gliadin's main purpose is to add consistency, chewiness, flavor, and protein. Gluten is also used in various household products, such as medications and skin lotions. The gluten in these products acts as a filler or binding agent.

But with all its positive contributions, gliadin can have serious consequences. In some people, gliadin can cause inflammation and the inability to absorb nutrients in the small intestine. These effects lead to autoimmune diseases such as celiac disease, osteoporosis, and arthritis. Other people experience less-intense reactions to gluten that still tend to affect their digestive systems.

Realizing how the differences between wheat and gluten affect your situation

You've probably seen the words *wheat-free* and *gluten-free* used interchangeably on food labels. But they're not interchangeable. Knowing the difference is essential when you start eliminating either one from your diet, for the following reasons:

- **You may have a specific condition that dictates what you cut from your diet.** You need to know why you're eliminating wheat, grains, gluten, or all of the above. Have you been diagnosed with celiac disease, are you allergic to wheat or grains, or are you gluten intolerant? (We focus on the answers to these questions in the rest of this chapter.)

- **To see results, you have to cut the right things.** A working knowledge of what you can eat is critical if you're going to be successful with your new lifestyle. This is especially important knowing that a reaction can occur with wheat/grains and not gluten, and vice-versa. The slightest amount of wheat, grains, or gluten left in a diet where it has been eliminated can be enough to prevent you from seeing the progress that you're hoping for.

✔ **You can save your sanity by knowing where the line is.** Making only necessary sacrifices can help you avoid becoming overwhelmed by this major life change. If you're giving up wheat or gluten but not all grains, understanding which items you can keep makes a diet change a little less daunting. That may sound silly now, but when you're cutting foods out of your diet, every little win counts. (If you're giving up gluten or grains, sorry; you have to give up all the wheat, too, as we explain later in the chapter.)

Checking Out Wheat-Related Allergies and Diseases

Your body may or may not be able to handle wheat, grains, and gluten. If you can't handle them, your body reacts in one of three ways:

✔ **Autoimmune disease:** Your body turns against itself and attacks healthy tissues. This is what happens with celiac disease in response to eating gluten. It can take anywhere from days to years for an autoimmune disease to develop.

✔ **Allergic reaction:** The immune system has an immediate reaction to something the body is hypersensitive to. The reaction can range from mild to immediate and potentially fatal.

✔ **Intolerance:** A food intolerance doesn't involve the immune system, and it's not life-threatening. It can take just a few minutes or several hours for your body to have an intolerance reaction. However, the symptoms may still be unpleasant.

We go into more detail about the differences between allergies and diseases in the following section. Then we explain the basics of celiac disease and wheat allergies and intolerance.

Relating wheat to allergies and diseases

An *allergy* is a bodily reaction to any substance that produces symptoms. Anything you eat, inhale, or touch can cause an allergy. Symptoms may include a runny nose, wheezing, asthma, hives, itchy eyes, constipation, diarrhea, or a skin rash. In regard to wheat, a wheat allergy produces symptoms within hours of eating wheat.

Wheat is a well-known allergen that leads to symptoms that are often attributed to other causes. If you suffer from allergies, eliminating wheat from your diet is the first step in identifying the source of your allergy.

To determine whether you're allergic to wheat, your doctor performs a physical exam, skin test, and blood test. He'll also likely ask you to complete a symptom questionnaire and keep a diary of your diet and symptoms. After you're diagnosed with a wheat allergy, you need to avoid all contact, ingestible and non-ingestible, with triggers associated with wheat.

Disease, on the other hand, is when your body doesn't function properly and you experience pain and/or physical discomfort. In the case of wheat- and grain-related diseases, gluten intolerance can cause celiac disease. Symptoms for celiac disease include abdominal cramping, diarrhea, vomiting, and weight loss.

Diseases have specific symptoms, but many symptoms can be the result of several, even dozens, of diseases. Symptomatically, celiac disease is often confused with other gastrointestinal disorders such as irritable bowel syndrome and food poisoning.

If you and your doctor suspect that you have celiac disease, you undergo blood tests and intestinal biopsies to identify the cause of symptoms. *Dermatitis herpetiformis,* also known as the *gluten rash,* can be used to confirm positive tests with the blood and biopsies.

After you're diagnosed with celiac disease, you'll probably feel relieved to know what's causing your symptoms and how to treat the disease. However, the only treatment known for celiac disease is total gluten-free living.

Understanding celiac disease

Celiac disease is a condition that damages the lining in the small intestine when you eat gluten. Celiac disease can be life-threatening for those who suffer from it.

Here's how it works: When you eat gluten (whether in wheat, barley, or rye), the immune system attacks the inner lining of your small intestine to prevent the gluten from being absorbed into the rest of your body and causing problems elsewhere. Pretty cool, huh? Yes, but when your immune system attacks the lining of the small intestines, the lining can't absorb anything else either, so malnutrition follows.

Symptoms of celiac disease can be hard to detect, but if you're experiencing some of the following symptoms, make an appointment with your doctor:

✔ Abdominal cramping and gas

✔ Achy joints

✔ Anemia

✔ Depression

✔ Diarrhea

✔ Fatigue

✔ Headaches

✔ Skin rashes

✔ Weight loss

If you suffer from celiac disease, the treatment is simple: Quit eating gluten. If you continue eating a gluten-rich diet, your body will be unable to absorb important vitamins and minerals. Continuing to eat gluten can lead to stunted growth, anemia, thyroid disease, osteoporosis, and cancer.

People diagnosed with celiac disease are better off than those people who suffer silently without symptoms. Celiac symptoms act as warning signals that something's not right. Those with no symptoms have no way of recognizing that they need to make changes and may unknowingly continue eating the foods that harm them.

We've presented a brief overview of celiac disease here. If you're diagnosed with the disease and want to know more about celiac and how to manage it, check out *Celiac Disease For Dummies* by Ian Blumer, MD, and Sheila Crowe, MD, and *Living Gluten-Free For Dummies* by Danna Korn (Wiley).

Identifying wheat intolerance versus wheat allergy

Wheat intolerances are much more common than wheat allergies. A *wheat intolerance* means your digestive system can't break down wheat-containing foods; it leads to gastric distress and other uncomfortable conditions. If you fall into the 15 to 20 percent of the U.S. population that suffers from wheat intolerance, you probably lack the enzymes necessary to break down wheat.

The symptoms of wheat intolerance are similar to the symptoms of other digestive system disruptions, making wheat intolerance difficult to diagnose. The symptoms can take hours to develop and days to go away, and you feel miserable the entire time. Symptoms of wheat intolerance include

- Constipation
- Diarrhea
- Eczema
- Fatigue
- Gas
- General aches and pains
- Headaches
- Mood swings
- Stomach bloating

Wheat allergies are a different story. Less than 1 percent of the U.S. population has an immediate allergic reaction to wheat consumption. Children are more commonly diagnosed with wheat allergies than adults are.

When you're allergic to wheat, your body mistakenly views one or more of the wheat proteins as something that's going to harm you. Your immune system produces antibodies to fight off the proteins, causing the allergic reaction. Symptoms include

- Abdominal cramps, nausea, and vomiting
- Anaphylaxis
- Asthma and restrictive breathing
- Coughing
- Diarrhea
- Hives
- Irritation of the mouth and throat
- Itchy and watery eyes
- Sinus congestion

An allergic reaction can occur in only a few minutes after you eat wheat. So if you suspect you're allergic to wheat, get tested by an allergist. A test for antibodies helps diagnose your wheat allergy and indicate where to go from there.

Although the situation is rare, wheat allergies can become life-threatening if anaphylaxis occurs. *Anaphylaxis* is an overreaction of your immune system to an allergen (in this case, wheat) that affects your whole body, possibly sending you into shock and causing labored breathing. If you have a family or personal history of anaphylaxis or other allergic reactions, you should always have two injectable doses of adrenaline (a common form is epinephrine) with you at all times. The symptoms of anaphylaxis affect people differently. This list includes all those symptoms so you know what to look out for:

- ✔ Breathing complications
- ✔ Change in skin color
- ✔ Chest pain
- ✔ Difficulty swallowing

- ✔ Dizziness
- ✔ Elevated heart rate
- ✔ Nausea and vomiting
- ✔ Skin rash

Comparing a Wheat- or Grain-Free Diet to a Gluten-Free Diet

When you're setting up your diet, you need to know what to look for specifically in regard to the condition you're treating. A wheat- or grain-free diet is just that: foods with no wheat or grain. Non-wheat grains with gluten, such as barley and rye, are okay if you're focusing only on wheat.

When planning a gluten-free diet, though, eliminating all grains containing gluten is critical. The following sections help you navigate what is and isn't still on your to-eat list and what other products you may need to avoid. You have to eliminate all wheat from your diet because you can't separate wheat and gluten. However, we suggest eliminating all grains, which automatically cuts out all gluten.

Knowing the foods to avoid

When making your don't-eat list for your new wheat-, grain- or gluten-free diet, you eliminate foods that may cause allergies and stomach problems. The following lists can help you design your diet to your liking.

Many non-wheat, non-gluten grains also contain the same problematic compounds as wheat. These compounds bind to a host of nutrients and block their absorption. These grains drive blood sugar spikes because of their carbohydrate content.

Grains to steer clear of on a wheat- or grain-free diet and a gluten-free diet are

- All forms of wheat
- Amaranth
- Barley
- Bran
- Couscous
- Durum
- Farina
- Farro
- Hemp
- Kamut
- Malt
- Millet
- Oats
- Orzo
- Quinoa
- Rice
- Rye
- Sorghum
- Spelt
- Teff
- Triticale

Wheat starch is wheat that has had its gluten washed out. The U.S. doesn't permit its use in gluten-free products because it's not believed to be totally free of gluten.

When it comes to foods that may or may not contain wheat/grains or gluten, you have to be vigilant. Unless the label says wheat- or grain-free or gluten-free, leave these foods out:

- Beer
- Breads
- Breakfast cereals
- Candy
- Condiments (such as ketchup, mustard, and mayonnaise)
- Cookies
- Crackers
- French fries
- Hot dogs
- Ice cream
- Pancakes
- Pasta
- Pastries
- Pizza crust
- Pretzels
- Processed meats
- Salad dressings
- Sauces
- Sausage
- Soups
- Soy sauce
- Waffles

Wheat can be found in many places, so if you eat foods that aren't included on this list, make sure to read the food label. (See Chapter 5 for more about food labels.)

Recognizing thumbs-up foods

Have you ever noticed that when you change your diet, the can't-have list of foods is always longer than the can-have list? Well, here's the good news: The can-have list for wheat-, grain-, and gluten-free eating isn't as restrictive as you may think. You can find plenty of good wheat/grain-free and gluten-free foods on the market, plus safe ingredients that let you turn out all kinds of goodies. (See Chapter 7 for more about stocking your kitchen; see Part III for healthy and tasty wheat- and grain-free recipes.)

All these foods are wheat/grain-free and gluten-free. Some of these foods may cause a rise in blood sugar, however, which leads to an insulin response. Foods on the can-have list include the following:

- All nonbreaded meat
- Dairy products (cream, milk, sour cream, lowfat Greek yogurt, and all cheese except for shredded cheese, unless it says "gluten-free")
- Eggs
- Fruits and vegetables
- Non-wheat flour (almond, arrowroot, buckwheat, cassava, chestnut, chia, coconut, flaxseed, potato, soy, and tapioca)

Unearthing hidden wheat and gluten

So you've tried everything you can think of to eliminate the wheat and gluten in your diet, but you're still suffering. Ah, what to do? Well, the first step is to make sure you haven't missed any less-than-obvious sources.

When looking to identify hidden wheat, always read the label. These key terms will surface when wheat is present:

- Contains wheat ingredients
- Dextrin
- Emulsifiers
- Flavorings and additives
- Hydrolyzed plant and vegetable protein
- Vegetable protein

Wheat and gluten can be found in other places where you may not think to look. For example, you may be ingesting or absorbing them through personal care products, appliances, and kids toys and art supplies. Go online to find a list of products that contain wheat and gluten so you know what to avoid. Or if you can't figure out whether your favorite beauty product contains wheat or gluten, call and ask the manufacturer about the ingredients in the product.

When treating celiac disease with a gluten-free diet, little wiggle room is available for cross-contamination. Gluten-free doesn't mean eliminating gluten just from your diet; it means removing it from your life. Consider the following items that can contain gluten:

- Art supplies (paint)
- Detergents (laundry and dishwasher)
- Hair conditioners
- Lipstick/lip balm
- Modeling compounds for kids (such as Play-Doh)
- Multiple-use paper plates, cups, and plasticware
- Nail polish
- Scratched or porous cookware and utensils where gluten can hide in the cracks
- Pots and pans that have been used to prepare foods containing gluten
- Shampoos
- Sunscreens
- Toasters and ovens used to prepare foods containing gluten

When it comes to your kitchen, make sure your cooking area is clean so food intended for someone who can't have wheat/gluten won't be cross-contaminated with the wheat and gluten in other foods.

Being aware of gluten replacements

When manufacturers remove gluten to create a gluten-free food, they also remove the wheat. In order for the food to maintain its structure, it must have a gluten replacement. These substitutes are various types of starches such as tapioca, rice, and potato. The binding and glueyness that these starches provide are adequate for most gluten-free people.

The starches that are added to give gluten-free food the needed binding and texture pose some alternative health risks. Basically, you trade gluten intolerance for elevated blood sugar and insulin levels, which lead to fat storage and diabetes. This swap presents another set of potential health issues, including Type 2 diabetes, heart disease, and cancer. Choosing alternative foods that don't contain these high starches is the best way to live gluten-free.

Chapter 4

Not the Whole-y Grail: Tracking Wheat's Relation to Overall Health

In This Chapter

▶ Understanding the process of metabolism

▶ Pulling the mask off so-called healthy whole grains

▶ Linking wheat consumption to leaky gut, inflammation, and other maladies

*P*robably the biggest obstacle to achieving success on a wheat-free lifestyle is wrapping your head around the fact that wheat isn't good for you. If you're in your 50s or younger, you've heard the "eat more grains and lower your fat intake" message for most of your life. Trying to delete that mindset from your brain's hard drive can be difficult.

Everyone is motivated to change by identifying what's most important to her. It can be a personal ailment or even a friend's poor health. It may be reaching what you consider middle age and not wanting to suffer the same fate as many around you. How many people do you know who suffer from arthritis, stomach issues, or neurological disorders such as dementia and Alzheimer's? These diseases are becoming more common despite a 50-year push that wheat is an essential part of a healthy diet. Something isn't working.

In this chapter, we hope to start the motivation process by explaining the negative health issues associated with wheat. We break down the process of digestion and then connect the dots to various disease states that are related to wheat consumption (even though they may not seem like it). Hopefully, a basic understanding of what is happening in your body after you eat the stuff will spur you to take control of your health.

Examining the Body's Response to Eating

Most people wake up every day and don't think twice about the multitude of complex processes taking place inside their bodies. So many of these processes are interrelated that the domino effect that can occur when one of them isn't working can be eye-opening. It all starts with the food you put in your mouth. Think of your body as a car and food as the gasoline. No matter how tuned up the car is, it won't run if you put in the wrong kind or wrong amount of gas.

So why does eating certain foods make people fat and lead to diabetes, heart disease, and obesity? Much of it has to do with metabolism, as we explain in the following sections.

Understanding how the body processes food

To understand how wheat affects your body, you need to understand how your body breaks down food, processes it, and distributes the resulting elements to be used as energy or stored for later use:

1. *Metabolism* begins when you eat food, which is made up of carbohydrates, fats, proteins, and fiber. Your stomach releases hydrochloric acid (HCL) to start to break down the food.

2. The partially broken-down food moves to the small intestine. Enzymes help break the food down even further. Proteins become amino acids; fats turn into fatty acids; and carbohydrates are converted into glucose and fructose (both forms of sugar). Fiber stays along for the ride, unfazed by what's going on around it. It helps keep the process moving but also limits the absorption of some of the nutrients in the food particles.

3. Amino acids, fatty acids, and sugars in the small intestine make their way to the liver. The liver takes as much as it can; any excess circulates throughout the body. At that point, the body (which keeps a very tight rein on how much glucose is allowed to circulate in the blood) tells the pancreas to increase insulin production.

4. Insulin now makes *glycogen* (the name for stored glucose) in the liver. It also directs amino acids from the bloodstream into the muscles, and the excess fatty acids are stored in the fat cells for future energy needs in the form of triglycerides.

Figure 4-1 shows the organs involved in digestion.

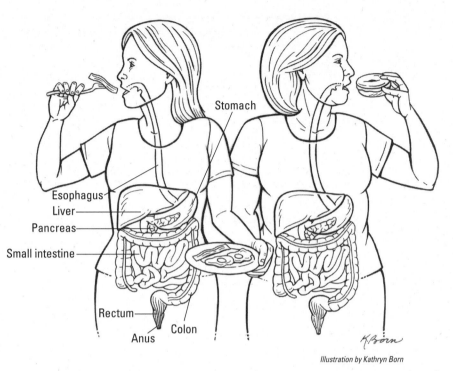

Figure 4-1:
The body processes a wheat-free diet differently than it processes a standard diet.

Stomach

Esophagus
Liver
Pancreas
Small intestine

Rectum
Anus
Colon

Illustration by Kathryn Born

Insulin, also known as the fat storage hormone, leads the glucose and fatty acids to fat cells that will take them. When you have stable blood sugar levels, insulin does this job easily and within normal ranges. However, when you eat carb-laden meals, the body is overwhelmed with glucose; the fat cells eventually quit responding to the knock on the door, so more and more insulin is required to perform the same task. This situation is the beginning of *insulin resistance.*

When insulin levels are high, the body tends to be in fat storage mode. When insulin levels are low, the body tends to be in fat purging mode (a state of using fat for energy).

A person who eats a wheat- or grain-free diet processes food differently than a person who eats an average diet filled with processed food, carbs, and sugar. Table 4-1 shows the comparison for the two women shown in Figure 4-1.

Table 4-1	Processing a Wheat-Free Diet vs. a Standard Diet
Wheat-Free Diet	**Standard Diet**
Because the woman on the left isn't carb dependent, she's satiated longer, requiring fewer meals and less thought about food throughout the day.	Because the woman on the right is carb dependent, she needs to eat every three to four hours to avoid a sugar crash. While thinking about eating carbohydrates, she begins secreting insulin.
She gets hungry and eats a meal free of wheat, grains, and added sugar.	She starts eating food containing wheat, grains, and added sugar.
Blood glucose, which has been stable all day, doesn't spike but slightly rises at a slow rate.	Blood glucose rises in the bloodstream quickly.
The pancreas releases a limited amount of insulin needed to clear glucose from the blood. Glucose levels return to baseline quickly.	The pancreas releases large amounts of insulin to clear the excess glucose from the blood.
Lack of insulin causes fat cells to release triglycerides for energy. She gets leaner.	Insulin transports the excess blood glucose to the fat cells for storage as triglycerides. She gets fatter.
In addition to her weight management, she won't develop leaky gut. Her risk for chronic illnesses such as heart disease, arthritis, dementia, Alzheimer's, and diabetes is reduced.	In addition to weight gain, she will likely develop leaky gut due to her inflammatory diet of wheat, grains, excess sugar, and vegetable oils.

Defining Type 1 and Type 2 diabetes

Type 1 diabetes, previously known as *juvenile diabetes* or *insulin dependent diabetes,* occurs when the pancreas can't produce the amount of insulin required to handle the sugar eaten. It's considered autoimmune in nature and is usually diagnosed in children and young adults. Type 1 diabetes comprises about 5 percent of all diabetes cases.

Type 2 diabetes, also known as *adult-onset or non-insulin dependent diabetes,* occurs when the pancreas either doesn't produce enough insulin or the body doesn't recognize the amount produced. This chronic condition makes up about 95 percent of diabetes cases and is considered preventable with proper diet.

Part of managing Type 1 diabetes is carefully monitoring carbohydrate intake. But people with Type 2 diabetes aren't told to lower their carbohydrate intake to keep insulin levels down. Rather, when fasting blood sugar levels get too high, doctors just put them on a drug to help contain the situation.

Storing fatty acids for later energy

When insulin asks cells to accept glucose and fatty acids for storage, it gets help from an enzyme called *lipoprotein lipase* (LPL). As insulin levels rise, so does LPL. Fatty acids are moved about in the bloodstream in the form of *triglycerides.* Triglycerides are too big to pass across the cell membrane, so LPL has the job of dismantling them into fatty acids and then reassembling them as triglycerides inside the cell, where they happily stay. Fat cells remain bloated until the triglycerides are called on for energy needs.

When insulin levels drop, so does LPL. Now the process is reversed, and an enzyme called *hormone-sensitive lipase* breaks down the triglycerides inside the cell so they can pass back through the cell membrane. This is a highly regulated process that functions to meet the body's energy needs.

Seeing how calories affect blood sugar levels

For far too long now, the message has been that all calories are created equal. Take in fewer calories than you burn, and you'll lose weight. And although that's partially true to some degree, it's not exactly the whole story. After insulin does its job and clears the glucose from the bloodstream, the resultant drop in blood sugar causes fatigue, brain fog, and moodiness until you eat again to bring blood sugar levels back up.

The term for this drop is *hypoglycemia,* and it's not a normal state for the body to be in. Most people who have hypoglycemia just accept it as part of who they are. However, hypoglycemia really indicates that the body isn't utilizing fat for energy and is too reliant on carbohydrates for fuel.

Eating a high-carb diet full of whole wheat just feeds the roller coaster of blood sugar swings. Rather than address the cause — what they're eating — people often opt to compensate by changing how often they're eating, moving to five or six small meals a day. But if you look at the *kind* of calories you're taking in, another solution becomes apparent. Taking in a given number of calories in the form of wheat causes rapid blood sugar spikes and drives you to eat again two to three hours later. Taking in the same number of calories in the form of fat elicits a slower and steadier blood sugar response that allows insulin to do its thing normally and lets stored body fat provide energy for hours on end. Satiation is achieved.

Hearing what the brain has to say about metabolism

As with most things with the body, the weight-gain picture is way more complex than just being the result of an abundance of insulin. Keeping glucose levels down allows insulin levels to stay low so the body dumps energy from the fat cells. But insulin levels can also rise in the absence of higher glucose levels. The culprit: a hormone called leptin.

Leptin is actually made by fat cells, a fact discovered only recently. Fat cells don't just lie around storing energy. The more fat cells you have, the more leptin is produced. Leptin acts as a messenger to the brain (mainly to the hypothalamus). The brain isn't able to monitor the body's energy balance, so it relies on leptin to act as its man in the field, so to speak. For a normal-weight person, the process goes as follows:

1. The person overeats and body fat levels go up. Consequently, leptin levels go up.

2. The brain gets the message and tells the body to reduce food intake and increase energy levels.

3. Body fat levels go down, leptin levels go down, and the brain tells the body to increase food intake and reduce energy levels.

With this system, the body maintains a stable weight, give or take a few pounds. (This consistency is also known as *homeostasis.*) But the situation is different for people who are overweight or obese:

1. The person overeats and body fat levels go up. Consequently, leptin levels go up.

2. The brain doesn't tell the body to reduce food intake. It thinks the person is still hungry, so she eats more and more and energy levels stay down.

In much the same way that the cells become resistant to insulin, the brain becomes resistant to leptin; more and more leptin is necessary to get the message across. Unfortunately, whereas the pancreas can create more insulin, you don't have an organ to produce more leptin. Only the fat cells can make it. Research has shown that this malady called *leptin resistance* may actually precede insulin resistance and weight gain itself.

Inflammation causes the brain to be less receptive to the leptin signaling. *Inflammation* is a very general term, however, so here are some of its various causes as it relates to leptin resistance:

- ✔ **Wheat, other grains, sugar, and refined food:** These foods, all of them carbohydrates, increase triglycerides. High triglycerides prevent leptin from passing through the blood-brain barrier. The leptin that does get through meets a weakened response due to the high fructose intake. (These foods can also lead to a condition called leaky gut, which we cover later in the chapter.)

- ✔ **Fatty acid imbalances:** You need an appropriate ratio of omega-6 fatty acids to omega-3 fatty acids in your diet. A ratio of 1:1 is most desirable, but the average American's ratio is closer to 15:1 or even 20:1. (See Chapter 18 for a more-detailed explanation.) The inflammation caused by this imbalance extends to the brain, disrupting leptin's message.

✔ **Stress and poor sleep:** Lack of sleep increases the stress hormone *cortisol,* which unleashes myriad negative effects. Stress and poor sleep can also work against your gut's stores of good bacteria.

✔ **Gut infections, food toxins, environmental toxins, and nutrient deficiencies:** All these factors contribute to leaky gut, which leads to inflammation and leptin resistance.

Debunking the Idea of Healthy Whole Grains

Say the words *whole grain,* and most people immediately think "healthy." That response is so ingrained (pardon the pun) in conventional wisdom that accepting a wheat-free lifestyle has to begin with a huge paradigm shift. Whole grains such as wheat are in no way healthy.

The United States Department of Agriculture (USDA) suggests six to eight servings per day of grains, with half of those coming from whole grains. Although most Americans still aren't reaching the whole-grain goal, whole-grain consumption has increased since the '90s. Yet diabetes and heart disease continue to be on the rise.

In the following sections, we take a look at wheat's nutritional content and the substances in wheat that can harm the body. (For details on gluten, head to Chapter 3.)

Defining whole and refined grain

Whole grain consists of three parts: the bran, the germ, and the endosperm:

✔ **Bran:** This outer layer of the grain kernel is mostly made of insoluble fiber. (The later section "Finding a replacement for wheat fiber" explains the difference between insoluble and soluble fiber.) Bran is removed in the milling process.

✔ **Endosperm:** *Endosperm* makes up the bulk of the seed weight. It's where white flour comes from.

✔ **Germ:** The *germ* is the part of the plant that sprouts to form a new plant. It's often removed in the milling process to make flour because its fat content, although low, can limit the product's shelf life.

Refined grains are what you get when the bran and germ are removed. Refining grains mills away most of the nutrients and fiber. Manufacturers enrich these foods to try to replace the lost nutrients, but they can't replace the fiber. That's why whole-grain foods are often advertised as being better than refined grains; many people assume the higher nutrient and fiber contents in whole grains are healthier. But fiber from wheat and other grains comes with its own health issues, as we discuss later in the chapter.

Looking at lectin's effects

The grains you eat are actually the seeds of the plant. The plant needs to propagate, but spreading its seed is much more difficult if an animal eats the seed before it can grow. Some plants, like roses or cacti, grow thorns to ward off predators. Wheat, on the other hand puts up a defense by creating substances called *lectins* that are toxic or *antinutritional* (inhibit nutrient absorption) to the creatures that eat it. (Don't confuse lectin and leptin. Lectin is found in plants and animals; leptin is a hormone in the body.) The seed passes through the digestive system intact, for the most part. After it passes out of the body, it survives to live another day.

Lectins are found in almost all plant and animal products in various amounts. Some of these include seeds, legumes, dairy products, potatoes, and tomatoes. Wheat and all other grains tend to have the highest concentrations. Lectin in wheat is particularly problematic because it's in the form of *wheat germ agglutinin* (WGA). This form, mostly concentrated in the seed, is able to withstand processes for combatting antinutrients (sprouting, fermentation, the general process of digestion, and so on). WGA is so tough, in fact, that its molecular structure is the same as human hair and vulcanized rubber!

WGAs are very small, and their tendency to accumulate in all types of tissues causes wide-ranging negative health effects, including (but not limited to) the following:

- ✔ **Damage to the intestinal wall:** This harm opens the door for all sorts of other issues (such as leaky gut, which we cover later in the chapter) that just ride the lectin's coattails through the openings in the gut wall.
- ✔ **Worsening insulin resistance and leptin resistance**
- ✔ **Neurotoxicity:** WGAs are able to cross the blood-brain barrier and inhibit *nerve growth factor,* a protein essential for proper brain function.

 WGAs aren't always the main cause of a disorder, but they're dangerous because of their ability to exacerbate a disease that is already present. The bottom line is to remove wheat or even all grains from your diet.

Finding a replacement for wheat fiber

Many people wonder whether they'll lack the required amount of fiber if they cut wheat and other grains from their diets. The short answer is "absolutely not!" In fact, some of the healthier foods you're replacing wheat with (vegetables and fruit) have more fiber than the fortified whole grains you were eating before.

Now for the bigger question: Do you need as much fiber as the recommendations say (25 to 40 grams per day)? Yes, but it shouldn't come from fortified grains whose effect hinders absorption of other nutrients.

To understand what fiber does for the body, you first have to differentiate between the types of fiber:

- ✔ **Soluble fiber:** *Soluble fiber* is considered *water soluble,* meaning it dissolves in water. It makes you feel full and slows down digestion because it expands in the gut. It also can produce sticky lumps in the intestine, which can lead to bloating and gas. Soluble fiber is more prone to fermentation, which helps feed the good bacteria in the gut. It's found in some vegetables, fruits, nuts, and legumes.

- ✔ **Insoluble fiber:** *Insoluble fiber* is not water soluble. It passes through the body mostly unchanged and tends to speed up transit time, if you will. It's not as prone to fermentation but may help spread the process of fermentation to the entire colon. Insoluble fiber is found in the skins of vegetables and fruits and the bran portion of whole grains.

Much of the research is inconclusive as to fiber's benefits. One of the biggest claims made for eating fiber is the increased time for digestion, which keeps blood sugar levels down (obviously an important benefit for diabetics). However, blood sugar levels decrease anyway on a wheat-free diet, so the need to slow digestion isn't as much of an issue.

Well-controlled studies shows no benefit from diets high in fiber for the reduction of colorectal cancer, diverticulitis, irritable bowel syndrome, or constipation. In reality, such a diet can worsen these conditions, despite what conventional wisdom would tell you.

Insoluble fiber in particular can have some additional consequences:

- ✔ **Leads to osteoporosis:** Because of the antinutritive effect, insoluble fiber inhibits the absorption of both calcium and zinc and depletes calcium the body already contains.

- ✔ **Increases vitamin deficiency diseases:** Because of the increase in transit time caused by insoluble fiber, your body doesn't absorb the fat soluble vitamins (A, D, E, and K) or phosphorus, iron, or magnesium as easily, which can lead to a variety of diseases.

High grain consumption leads to more health problems

Modern man has become completely dependent on cereal grains, with 56 percent of the food energy and 50 percent of the protein consumed on earth coming from eight cereal grains. Wheat is number one.

In more than half the countries of the world, bread provides more than 50 percent of the total caloric intake. In many developing countries, grains are the predominant food staple — the only thing keeping people from starving to death. But even where hunger is no longer the main problem, malnourishment is still common. And it's often accompanied by obesity and diabetes. That may seem like a paradox, but as we explain in Chapter 2, the staff of life can be anything but.

The takeaway is to eat soluble fiber from fruits, vegetables, and fermented foods and don't sweat trying to go overboard with your fiber intake. Follow the tenets of this book, and you shouldn't have to give any extra thought to adding or supplementing with extra fiber.

Recognizing wheat's vitamin and mineral shortcomings

The problem with eating a diet high in wheat and grains is that they squeeze out calories and nutrients from other foods without fully replacing them. The nutrients in milled/processed grains have low *bioavailability,* which means the body can't access and absorb them. Even unrefined grains are limited by the toxins the plant produces to fend off predators.

Plants are equipped with antinutrients called gluten, lectins, and phytates. Some animals can handle the toxins, but humans can't. *Gluten,* of course, causes intolerance-related symptoms in many people, even those who don't have full-blown celiac disease. Lectins bind to insulin receptors and the intestinal lining, causing GI distress (as explained earlier in the chapter). *Phytates* can bind to minerals and slow their absorption.

To see what we mean, check out the following list of vitamin and mineral quantities in wheat and grains:

- **Vitamin A:** None in grains. Only yellow maize contains beta carotene, which the body converts to vitamin A. Lack of vitamin A is a huge problem in developing countries because of their high wheat consumption; there, this deficiency is a major determining factor for childhood disease and mortality. Vitamin A deficiency exacerbates infectious disease symptoms.

✔ **Vitamin B:** Vitamin B12 is found in animal products only. Generally, grains contain the rest of the B vitamins, but their bioavailability isn't very high. For example, whereas your body can utilize 100 percent of the B6 available in meat, it can access only 20 to 25 percent of the amount in wheat. Vitamin B12 deficiency hinders the production of red blood cells, nerves, and DNA. Lack of other B vitamins, such as thiamine, riboflavin, and niacin, leads to all kinds of problems, including reproductive problems and the inability to synthesize insulin.

✔ **Vitamin C:** None. Vitamin C is important for your bones, skin, and connective tissue, especially in the area of wound healing.

✔ **Vitamin D:** None naturally. Many cereals are fortified with vitamin D. Lack of this vitamin contributes to rickets and poor bone health and may be a player in the development of diabetes, multiple sclerosis, and hypertension.

✔ **Vitamin E:** None to speak of in wheat, with minimal amounts in other grains. Vitamin E deficiency contributes to neurological issues, gastrointestinal diseases, and reproductive issues.

✔ **Calcium:** Very little. These low amounts combined with high levels of phosphorus and magnesium in wheat lead to increased calcium loss and thus bone loss.

✔ **Iron:** Very little, which is a major issue because iron deficiency is the most common nutritional problem in the world, affecting about 30 percent of the population. Getting too little of this vitamin leads to fewer red blood cells and less oxygen throughout the body.

✔ **Zinc, copper, and magnesium:** Very little of all three, resulting in decreased immune function and, in the case of magnesium, increased risk of heart disease and diabetes as well as muscle weakness and personality changes.

Getting to Know Leaky Gut

Gut permeability, also known as *leaky gut,* started out as just a theory in the alternative medicine crowd but has since been proven to be a real and measurable syndrome. Science is still trying to figure out the ins and outs of the whole process, which is one reason many doctors are slow to (or fail to) recognize and diagnose leaky gut. In the following sections, we explain how your gut works — well, doesn't work — when leaky gut rears its head, and we lay out some symptoms you may not realize are tied to this condition.

Surveying what goes wrong with your gut

Understanding leaky gut may seem like a daunting task, but it really isn't. Think about your bathroom shower lined with porcelain tiles and grout. The tiles and grout have to be impenetrable to protect the space behind them. Otherwise, mold and rot can occur over time unless you catch the problem early and seal the grout before the full extent of the damage is realized.

Now apply this imagery to your gut. Your shower tiles are now the outer layers of your intestinal cells, also known as *epithelial cells,* which absorb nutrients. The epithelial cells allow only desirables (such as properly broken-down nutrients from food) to pass. The spaces between the epithelial cells are called the *tight junctions* (see Figure 4-2); their job is to fill the space between the cells that are working to absorb the proper nutrients. Like the grout around the bathroom tile, the tight junctions are supposed to be impermeable.

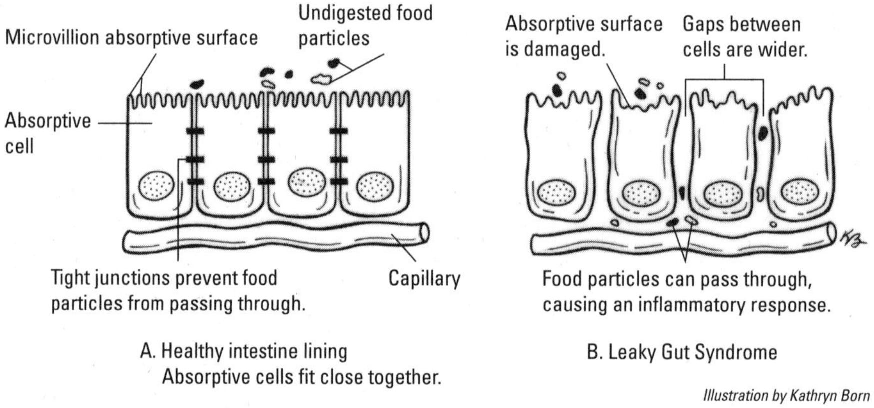

Figure 4-2:
Tight junctions aren't always as tight as they should be.

Microvillion absorptive surface

Undigested food particles

Absorptive cell

Tight junctions prevent food particles from passing through.

Capillary

A. Healthy intestine lining
Absorptive cells fit close together.

Absorptive surface is damaged.

Gaps between cells are wider.

Food particles can pass through, causing an inflammatory response.

B. Leaky Gut Syndrome

Illustration by Kathryn Born

However, certain external factors such as wheat, stress, and antibiotics can trigger the tight junctions to fall asleep on the job over time. The discovery of a protein called zonulin in 2000 made scientists realize the tight junctions weren't so tight. Just like bathroom grout can wear away over time and provide less protection from invaders, so too can the tight junctions get to the point of permeability. After they're compromised, the tight junctions actually open like doors and let undesirables such as undigested food, toxins, and other waste into the bloodstream.

The chain reaction that follows goes something like the following:

1. The tight junctions fail to stay closed, and they allow undesirables to pass through and into the bloodstream.

2. The liver tries to filter the unintended guests but is overwhelmed by the flow of pathogens, toxins, and undigested food.

Alessio Fasano: Cracking the code of leaky gut

Alessio Fasano is the man responsible for discovering the protein zonulin. As we describe in this chapter, zonulin is integral to leaky gut and autoimmune disease. With this discovery, Fasano opened up a world of treatment that shifted the emphasis to the intestines and away from just treating the symptoms of various individual maladies. However, in doing so, he implicated gluten-filled grains such as wheat as a major culprit.

Fasano points to three things that need to be present for many diseases such as celiac or autoimmune conditions to set in. They are

✔ A genetic predisposition to a particular disease.

✔ An environmental factor that starts the immune response.

✔ A way to cross the safety barriers that the body has set up to prevent certain diseases from doing their damage. In the case of celiac disease and autoimmune conditions, that crossing is leaky gut. In essence, the leaky gut allows the first two factors to work together.

Unfortunately, celiac disease is the only disease for which scientists currently know the environmental trigger. And of the three factors, only the genetic disposition is completely out of your control.

3. Realizing that dangerous invaders are escaping, your immune system does its best to eliminate the invaders, but it's overwhelmed as well.

4. The invaders roam the body at will and settle in various tissues, leading to inflammation in those particular areas.

5. The immune system is now on red alert and working on all cylinders just to keep up with its normal duties (defending the gut, cleaning the blood, and warding off pathogens) in addition to dealing with the localized inflammation. Autoimmune conditions can follow.

Knowing the symptoms of and treatments for leaky gut

Leaky gut can be difficult to get diagnosed because its symptoms are wide ranging and can seem unrelated to each other. Here's a partial list of ailments that may be signs of leaky gut (and we emphasize the word *partial*):

✔ Autoimmune diseases such as celiac, rheumatoid arthritis, Type 1 diabetes, and multiple sclerosis

✔ Chronic diarrhea and constipation

✔ Chronic fatigue and muscle pain

✔ Depression and anxiety

✔ Frequent sickness

✔ Inflammatory bowel disease

✔ Migraine headaches, brain fog, and memory loss

✔ Multiple food sensitivities

✔ Nutrient deficiencies

✔ Obesity and Type 2 diabetes

✔ Skin conditions such as psoriasis and eczema

Treating these and other leaky gut symptoms individually is like just slapping a bandage on a gaping wound. In order to truly eliminate the symptoms, you have to treat the underlying cause. If you or your doctor thinks leaky gut may be the root of one or more of your symptoms, you can do a few basic things to address it:

✔ **Cut the wheat.** *Gliadin,* one of the two main proteins in wheat gluten, causes an increase in zonulin. Elevated levels of zonulin cause the tight junctions and the blood-brain barrier to allow invaders through for a period of a few hours to a few days. Removing wheat from your diet helps reduce your zonulin levels.

✔ **Take refined carbohydrates, sugar, and processed foods out of your diet.** The chemicals and preservatives in these foods cause gut inflammation because your body wasn't built to handle them, especially in the quantities that most people take in. Refined sugar can also lead to an overgrowth of bacteria and yeast, another cause of leaky gut. Eliminating sugar starves the bacteria overgrowth so it can't propagate.

✔ **Reduce your use of antibiotics, NSAIDS, aspirin, and prescription hormones like birth control pills.** Part of what makes the gut susceptible to inflammation and leakage is an imbalance in the bacteria in the gut. Certain medications kill off not only the bad bacteria but also the good bacteria (a condition called *dysbiosis.*) The bacteria colonies aren't able to keep each other in check, and the bad ones have a chance to flourish. NSAIDS and aspirin in particular irritate the stomach lining, leading to more inflammation and permeability.

After long-term antibiotic use, taking probiotics helps restore the bacteria balance in your gut (because your gut can't do so on its own). Adding fermented foods to your diet will do double duty, along with the probiotics, toward healing your gut bacteria.

✔ **Rid yourself of chronic stress.** That ache you feel in your belly from stressful situations is a reminder of the link between the brain and the stomach. The occasional pregame or prespeech jitters don't cause a huge problem, but sustained stress over time creates continual gut damage, paving the way for a suppressed immune system, inflammation, and gut leakage. Steps to eliminate stress include exercising; practicing breathing techniques, mindfulness, and/or meditation; and expressing gratitude.

✔ **Eliminate chronic infections.** Much like chronic stress, chronic infections cause an environment that paves the way for a bacterial imbalance in the gut. Although a wheat-free lifestyle can't guarantee you'll never have another infection, adhering to the principles we discuss throughout this book can help you avoid chronic infection.

Tying Wheat to Other Health Conditions

The negative effects of wheat consumption are wide ranging. We discuss its part in gut damage earlier in the chapter, but in the following sections, we explain how eating wheat can impact your heart, brain, and skin.

Exploring wheat's role in heart disease

Many people are surprised to learn that wheat, sugar, and vegetable oils play a part in the lead-up to heart disease. Specifically, they contribute to *metabolic syndrome,* a conglomeration of disorders that are very strong indicators for heart disease.

Inflammation and oxidative damage are the true causes of heart disease, but some easily measurable markers can tell you whether you're on the road to trouble. Metabolic syndrome, also known as syndrome X, is made up of five characteristics that are risk factors for developing heart disease when at least three of them occur together. The "official" list varies minimally among different organizations, but for our purposes we use the American Heart Association's (AHA's) guidelines:

✔ **Elevated waist circumference:** This factor is the broadest because so many things go into making someone overweight. However, as we note earlier in the chapter, insulin and leptin levels contribute to weight gain, and wheat's and sugar's effect on these levels is undeniable. Limit these foods and maintain a fairly constant blood glucose level, and bodyweight should remain stable.

To measure your waist circumference, wrap a tape measure around the top of your hipbones. After a normal gentle exhale, gently tighten the tape. If your measurement is more than 40 inches (for men) or 35 inches (for women), you have elevated waist circumference.

✔ **High fasting triglycerides:** *Triglycerides* are fats made by your liver. The AHA threshold indicates that levels at or above 150 are high, though we think that figure should probably be closer to 100. The only way to achieve low triglyceride levels is with a wheat-free, low-sugar, low-carbohydrate, and high-fat diet. For an explanation of triglycerides and how to find out what your levels are, refer to Chapter 17.

✔ **Low HDL:** *HDL* is a type of protein that moves the good cholesterol around in your body. You want this number to be high, so the AHA considers numbers lower than 40 (men) and 50 (women) to be risk factors. (We consider these thresholds the bare minimum. Ideally, we'd like to see those numbers bumped to at least 50 and 60, respectively.)

As you've probably guessed, wheat and vegetable oils contribute to lower HDL numbers. Fat, especially the healthy saturated fat found in grass-fed meats and butter, can raise your HDL number; it steadily continues to rise to between 80 and 90 for many people that maintain a wheat-free diet higher in healthy fats. Exercise contributes to an increase in this number as well, but not as much as diet does. Chapter 17 has more information on HDL levels and their connection to wheat.

✔ **High blood pressure:** Higher blood pressure causes stress on the arterial walls, which can lead to damage and heart disease. What constitutes "high"? Levels at or above 135/85. Cutting the grains and added sugar, including highly refined processed foods, naturally lowers blood pressure by decreasing the kidneys' salt absorption (though in some cases, it does such a good job you may actually need to add some iodized salt back into your diet).

✔ **High fasting glucose:** The AHA lists fasting glucose levels at or above 100 as "high," though we feel a number somewhere in the 80s is a better goal. Years and years of eating grains and sugar increases blood glucose levels. The body does an inadequate job of handling the excess glucose to the point that even after fasting, levels remain high.

All the risk factors contained in metabolic syndrome are just that — risk factors. They don't tell you whether you definitely will or won't get heart disease. They simply indicate whether your lifestyle puts you at a dramatically increased risk for heart disease.

Connecting grains to brain inflammation

In the earlier section "Knowing the symptoms of and treatments for leaky gut," we describe how wheat consumption can increase levels of zonulin, which causes the blood-brain barrier to allow unwanted particles through and leads to inflammation. Science has shown a link between this inflammation and neurological diseases such as Parkinson's, Alzheimer's, and dementia (in addition to neurological symptoms of leaky gut such as migraines and brain fog).

The brain contains 100 billion *neurons,* or nerve cells, and something like 1 to 5 trillion glial cells. *Glial cells* are involved in a number of processes, including inflammation. After these cells become inflamed, they stay that way; they don't have an off switch. They tend to cause the surrounding neuron cells to die off.

All the suspects that result in leaky gut are suspects for brain inflammation: wheat, other grains, sugar, processed foods, NSAIDS, antibiotics, aspirin, stress, and chronic infections. Environmental toxins play a role as well.

One of the best indicators for future dementia or Alzheimer's is a high fasting glucose level or high hemoglobin A1C (see Chapter 17). As you eat wheat and sugar, the high blood glucose can bind to proteins, causing an increase in free radicals and inflammation. And although some free radicals are necessary for life, too many of these fellows can cause serious neurological and other problems.

A blood glucose spike isn't the only risk factor wheat poses. The gluten in wheat provides another inflammatory trigger in the form of *cross-reactivity*. In this process, the unwanted gluten molecule that has entered the bloodstream resembles a molecule of neurological tissue, so while the autoimmune response is attacking gluten it also mistakenly attacks brain tissue.

Realizing acne isn't just skin deep

When you hear "acne," you probably have the image of a hormonal teenager with skin issues. However, adult-onset acne, especially in women, is extremely common. Topical ointments, creams, or even an oral antibiotic can treat the symptoms, but ultimately they're only temporary solutions. The long-term answer is (surprise!) linked to your gut health. After all, the skin is a mirror to what's happening inside the body; it's not immune to the inflammation that occurs internally.

The gastrointestinal (GI) mechanism correlates with and skin conditions such as acne (as well as other maladies such as depression and anxiety). In fact, research has shown that the adolescents with acne are more likely to suffer from GI symptoms such as constipation, halitosis, bloating, and gastric reflux.

Inflammation isn't the only wheat-related trigger; insulin spikes can cause acne as well. When you consume wheat, your body produces more insulin to counteract the rise in blood sugar. The increases in insulin cause the body to secrete an excess of the oily substance *sebum,* which rises to the surface of the skin through the pores. Normal amounts of sebum provide a protective barrier against bacterial and fungal infections. Excess amounts, however, lead to clogged pores and acne.

Part II

Making Wheat-Free Your Dietary Foundation

Five Categories of Vegetables to Include in a Wheat-Free Diet

- **Dark, leafy greens** such as spinach, kale, and collard and mustard greens
- **Brightly colored vegetables** such as peppers, carrots, and eggplant
- **Root vegetables** such as sweet potatoes, radishes, and beets
- **Cruciferous vegetables** such as broccoli, cabbage, cauliflower, bok choy, and Brussels sprouts
- **Other non-starchy vegetables** such as onions, cucumbers, celery, and mushrooms (okay, mushrooms are technically a fungus)

 When you alter your diet to exclude wheat, grains, sugar, and oil, you move through a change process, which can be described by the acronym DISCOVERY. To find out what the letters stand for, see the free article at www.dummies.com/extras/livingwheatfree.

In this part...

- Identify the reasons you want to go wheat- or grain-free and form a plan to meet your goal.

- See how a wheat/grain-free diet fits with other popular diets.

- Take a look at what's truly important on a food label and use that knowledge to clean out and restock your kitchen for your new healthy lifestyle.

Chapter 5

Eliminating Wheat from Your Diet for Good

So you're ready to make a change in your life by getting rid of wheat in your diet but aren't quite sure how to go about making the change last. Never fear; the change process isn't so dreadful after all. By answering certain questions and discovering what you really want, you can be better equipped to set goals that will propel you into eating a wheat-free, grain-free diet. (Although our primary focus is on eliminating wheat, we also advocate cutting all grains from your diet because they often have similar effects on your body.)

In this chapter, we help you begin to identify the challenges that change presents and figure out where you are in the change process. We explain the different stages of change and give you the tools necessary to help move forward with each stage. Finally, we show you how to write effective goals for your new wheat-free lifestyle.

Facing the Challenges Associated with Going Wheat-Free

Change is tough, especially when it comes to your diet. How many times have you set out to modify your food intake only to see your good intentions crash and burn because of an obstacle you weren't prepared for? Having an alternate plan in place is planning for success.

Most people fall into two common traps when trying to make a dietary change (wheat-free, grain-free, or otherwise). First, they wait to be motivated by something external, like a doctor or spouse telling them to lose weight. Second, they try to manufacture a motivator, like telling themselves they should eat better to be healthier. But these approaches often fail to motivate because they feel like chores; being told to change their behavior often makes people automatically put up a wall of resistance. True motivation comes when you make the decision to change on your own because it's important to you right now.

Another major challenge of going wheat-free is the withdrawal symptoms you may experience. Other obstacles include food itself, your thoughts and emotions about your new diet, and your behavior toward food. We explore all these challenges in the following sections.

Knowing what withdrawal symptoms you'll face

For some, one of the biggest difficulties in kicking the wheat habit is overcoming its addictive qualities. *Gliadin,* a wheat-containing protein, is broken down in the digestive tract into substances called exorphins. *Exorphins* are protein particles that come from outside of the body (from substances such as food and heroin) and masquerade as *endorphins* (natural substances in the body that cause feelings of euphoria and happiness). The exorphins bind to the same opiate receptors in the brain that endorphins do, leading to the same physical and emotional feelings. When you remove wheat from your diet, the exorphins cease to bind to these receptors, leading to a state of withdrawal. While this withdrawal is occurring, the body experiences a shift from *glycogen metabolism,* when your body is primarily burning glucose (sugar) for energy, to fat metabolism, where it "learns" to mobilize fat stores for energy.

Many people experience no withdrawal symptoms, but others have negative feelings that can last from one to four weeks. When this period ends, mental clarity and energy improve and appetite and cravings decrease. The following symptoms are associated with wheat withdrawal:

- ✔ Anxiety
- ✔ Constant hunger
- ✔ Depression
- ✔ Diarrhea
- ✔ Dizziness

- ✔ Fatigue
- ✔ Irritability
- ✔ Lack of energy
- ✔ Lightheadedness
- ✔ Mental fogginess
- ✔ Nausea
- ✔ Stomach cramps
- ✔ Strong cravings for wheat

Although the withdrawal symptoms from wheat elimination aren't devastating, they're still quite uncomfortable for some. If you're one of the unfortunate people who experience some of these symptoms, seeing the detoxification process through till the end may be challenging for you. The temptation to return to eating wheat in order to avoid the symptoms of withdrawal can be overwhelming. The good news is that if you've reached this withdrawal point, then you've clearly shown a desire to make a change. This desire feeds the purpose of your change and therefore increases your motivation.

Addressing challenges presented by food

The most obvious challenge in adopting a wheat-free lifestyle is to stop eating the countless foods that contain wheat. Here are the obstacles you have to face:

- ✔ **Food addictions and carbohydrate cravings:** The addictive qualities of wheat pose unique challenges for eliminating it from your diet.

    We suggest a cold-turkey approach when eliminating wheat from your diet. The weaning process prolongs the agony of addictions and cravings and further complicates the removal process.

- ✔ **Incorrect dietary information:** You're less likely to commit to a wheat-free diet if you lack the information necessary to change. For several decades, the mandate has been that eating a diet of whole wheat or whole grains is healthy. MyPlate, the U.S. guidelines for dietary intake, illustrates that you should get the majority of your calories from grains. Educating yourself on the harmful effects of wheat and other grains (see Chapter 4) can help you stay the course of your new lifestyle.

- ✔ **The convenience of the wheat-filled fast-food industry:** Lots of fast-food options contain wheat (and we're not just talking about the buns). The ease and expediency of these wheat-containing foods has created several generations of increased obesity, Type 2 diabetes, heart disease, and cancer. Other convenience foods outside the fast-food industry are also filled with wheat; from deli meats and veggie patties to salad dressings and fried fish sticks, wheat is prevalent throughout the convenience food market.

✔ **The grocery bill:** Yes, eating a wheat-free, whole-food diet is more expensive than eating the cheaper grain products you've been buying. No, you don't have to break the bank to eat wheat-free.

Whenever possible, purchase raw ingredients instead of buying prepared foods; raw foods are usually less expensive. Also, certain cuts of meat are cheaper than others. Purchase the more affordable ones so you don't grow to resent your new diet. Flip to Chapter 7 for more guidance on shopping for wheat-free foods.

Revamping your thoughts and emotions

You've probably had the same thoughts and beliefs about food for most of your life. Changing your mindset toward food — especially when you're eliminating something that feels like a staple in your diet — is tough, no doubt about it. Here are some ways to overcome the mental and emotional challenges that come with going wheat-free:

✔ **Set goals.** Your vision and goals are the skeletal system of the change process. Without these key components, your plan has no structure.

✔ **Be confident.** If you believe that you can accomplish a goal, you're more likely to work harder at it.

Several ways to increase your confidence include recalling past successful experiences and the strengths they required, setting easily obtainable goals, and identifying strategies to help you get what you want.

✔ **Take control of your food and lifestyle choices.** What you choose to eat is your decision. Period. Consciously making wheat-free choices may not always be easy, especially when doing so goes against what you're used to, but it's a key to your success.

Food choices are only part of a healthy lifestyle. Running yourself ragged, not getting enough sleep, and stressing out aren't conducive to your new way of living. Remove the clutter and drama from your life so you can make room for big, healthy changes.

✔ **Deal with your emotional eating habits.** Lots of people are emotional eaters; they eat to celebrate happiness, calm anger or stress, and soothe sadness. The stronger the emotion, the more profound the effect. And many foods people turn to for emotional eating contain wheat.

If you don't acknowledge your emotions and how they can direct your behavior, you're missing out on the powerful influence they have on your ability to change. Identifying what you're emotionally feeling and meeting those needs in a healthier way helps you fight the temptation to be emotional eaters.

✔ **Evaluate your readiness and willingness to change.** Removing wheat and other grains from your diet is a huge endeavor; it's one well worth it, but if you feel you can't put in the time or effort necessary right now, you may need to examine whether this is the right time to make such a fundamental change in your life. If it isn't, decide when will be. (We're talking about when in the short-term future here; deciding to fit going wheat-free into your five-year plan isn't going to improve your lifestyle.)

Modifying your actions

Your actions follow your thoughts. After you begin to change how you think about food, you'll find it easier to change your behaviors. Here are some behavioral changes that can help you shift into your wheat-free lifestyle:

✔ **Journal your progress.** A journal allows you to measure your progress, analyze your food intake, and keep your wheat-free goals in the forefront of your thinking. As you journal your food intake, you become aware of exactly what you're eating.

✔ **Break non-wheat-free routines.** When you drop wheat and grains from your diet and substitute those foods with noncarbohydrate foods, you become more satiated with less food, meaning you may need to eat less frequently. One routine that can be very difficult to get out of is consuming three square meals a day with a snack or two in between. In a wheat-free diet, needing only a couple of meals a day isn't uncommon.

✔ **Create an environment conducive to a wheat-free lifestyle.** Change is hard enough without the added stress of feeling like your surroundings are throwing up roadblocks every step of the way. Rid your kitchen completely of wheat products (as we detail in Chapter 7) and remove all triggers from your daily routine to minimize strain on your efforts to make a lasting change in your diet. Make sure you have a support system in place; family members or friends who sabotage your efforts (intentionally or otherwise) can make the process that much more difficult.

Find an accountability buddy. As we discuss in the later section "Maintaining accountability," having someone to hold you accountable helps solidify your commitment and strengthens your personal responsibility to the goals you've set.

Tackling the Change Process

One decision can change your life forever. Hopefully, the health consequences of a wheat-filled diet have piqued your interest in a lifestyle change (see Chapter 4 for more details).

The motivation to change is a simple process with a challenging plan of action that differs from person to person. Your beliefs, attitudes, and values play a huge part in the types of behaviors you engage in. They all contribute to what matters most to you in any given area of your life, especially your diet. Changing to a wheat-free diet requires mental and behavioral preparations that we outline in the following sections.

Identifying where you are in the change process

The Stages of Change Model by Prochaska, Norcross, and DiClemente provides insight into the inner workings of the change process. The following list outlines the stages of change and gives you some specific tools you can use to help you move to the next level.

- **Precontemplation:** This stage is characterized by two different groups:

  - The "I can't change" phase, where people have tried unsuccessfully in the past to change a behavior and don't believe they're capable of successfully changing now

  - The "I won't change" phase, where people don't believe that their current behavior is harmful

  In both cases, the cons outweigh the pros to the point of inaction. Setting small and easily obtainable goals that boost your confidence level and gathering information about the benefits of cutting wheat out of your diet can help push you into the next stage.

- **Contemplation:** This stage is highlighted by the people in the "I might change" phase. They're ambivalent about the modifications that they're considering making and the benefits of establishing new, healthier dietary choices. Some people can stay in this stage for months or even years.

- **Preparation:** This stage belongs to people in the "I will change" phase. Typically, they're planning to execute a change within the next six months. They often make small, subtle changes as a way to test the waters and build confidence before a larger, more desirable change takes place.

- **Action:** This stage is the "I am" phase. It's defined by the first six months of change to the new, wheat-free diet. During this stage, people are developing new habits and creating routines. This stage comes with a high risk of lapse and relapse, so having a plan of action for the obstacles that you'll encounter is critical. Making a deeper commitment to yourself by telling others of your change, having an accountability buddy to report to, and planning how to handle future obstacles are effective ways to keep the ball rolling and your motivation high.

✔ **Maintenance:** Congratulations! You've made it to the top of the mountain in the quest for eliminating wheat from your diet (give yourself a pat on the back). This stage is marked by being wheat-free for more than six months and is also known as the "I am still" phase. The key at this point is to stay here. You can accomplish this task by becoming a role model for others and creating an environment around them that is conducive for success, such as a wheat-free kitchen.

Don't get complacent after you reach the maintenance stage; it's still a time to be very careful of relapse.

You constantly move in and out of the various stages of the process depending on your current circumstances. For example, maybe you're in the maintenance stage with your wheat-free diet when along comes a two-week vacation that totally disrupts your eating pattern. You may then need to back up a few steps to the preparation or contemplation stage to get things back on track.

Implementing tools that lead to lasting change

Few people can decide to change and then just do it. You'll probably want to find ways to stay motivated to increase your chances of success with a wheat- or grain-free diet. We suggest applying the following techniques because your behavior begins with your thought processes.

Working your way from willpower to discipline

A lot of times, people claim they don't have the willpower to take on a drastic change like going wheat- or grain-free, but the truth is that no one makes such a shift on willpower alone.

Willpower is doing what you think you should do. Research shows that willpower is like a gas tank; as you exert willpower throughout the day, your tank gets lower and lower until you run out of fuel and can't resist going back to your old ways. But as you strengthen your willpower over time, you begin to gain self-control. You're able to do what you know is the right thing to do even when you feel a small degree of resistance. Eventually, you become disciplined.

Both willpower and self-control generate a have-to or should-do mentality, where you have little actual desire to perform the new behavior. _Discipline_ involves very little thought; you simply do what needs to be done without having to psych yourself up to make that choice.

By generating positive thinking in the form of mindfulness, expressed gratitude, and positive self-talk, you're better equipped to handle the challenges that eliminating wheat from your diet presents. You can use each tool by itself or together to form an unbeatable combination. Whichever approach you choose, it all starts with your frame of mind.

Practice mindfulness

When was the last time you drove across town, reached your destination, and then asked yourself, "How in the world did I get here?" Have you ever been so lost in thought that the conversation you were having with your spouse went in one ear and out the other? Do you ever look down at your plate and barely recall eating any of the food that's suddenly not there?

If so, you're not alone. Lots of people live life on autopilot and miss out on so much that life has to offer. This rut is where your health, and more specifically your diet, suffers. You lose sight of day-to-day self-care practices because you give your attention to other issues.

So how can you breakout of this pattern? *Mindfulness* is the nonjudgmental awareness of the present moment. In essence, it's stopping and smelling the roses. It requires focus, attention, and patience; you have to quiet all the voices and noises in your head and pay close attention to what's happening in the moment. When you practice mindfulness, your appreciation grows for the object of your focus. This practice is what helps answer the questions, "What's most important to me right now?" and "What do I need right now?"

As you make the switch to a wheat-free diet, become more mindful of the food you're eating. For example, take a bite-sized piece of meat. Look at it very carefully: What do you see? What color is it? What shape is it? Write down every nonjudgmental (that is, objective) word you can think of to describe what it looks like. Then write down every word you can think of that describes its smell. Do the same to describe its feel (both in your hands and on your tongue) and its taste. Describe all of the sensations that you're experiencing.

Considering all the changes that you have to make to go wheat-free can be overwhelming. However, the more you practice mindfulness, the more confidence you gain in switching to a wheat-free diet.

Express gratitude

When was the last time you expressed gratitude for something someone did for you? How often do you find yourself communicating gratefulness? Expressing gratitude generates positive emotions each time you thank someone because your focus is on the good of the other person, not yourself. The real benefits come when you live your life with an attitude of gratitude.

This positive approach to life doesn't mean that you look at life from a Pollyanna mindset or that you ignore life's difficult times. Instead, it's a realistic viewpoint of your abilities and an optimistic approach to life's challenges. Positive thinking also makes you more resilient, allowing you the strength to address adversity head-on. What does gratitude have to do with eliminating wheat from your diet? It provides the positive thinking and resiliency necessary for you to succeed in the change process. These tools come in quite handy when the challenges of change test your commitment level.

Engage in positive self-talk

The conversations you have with yourself — your *self-talk* — greatly affect your outlook on life and level of motivation. A quick analysis of your behaviors reflects the types of dialogues you have with yourself. Your beliefs dictate the direction of your self-talk, which is why positive self-talk generates the confidence needed to do your best and negative self-talk creates the self-doubt that often leads to failure. Here's how you can use self-talk to encourage your wheat-free shift:

- **Understand the power of self-talk.** Thoughts lead to beliefs, beliefs lead to feelings, and feelings lead to actions. By appreciating the strengths of both positive and negative self-talk, you're better able to put each in its rightful place and move forward with your behavior.

- **Focus on your positive beliefs.** This focal point includes the positive benefits of performing a particular behavior and the positive belief that you have the ability to succeed with the behavior. The idea is based on the belief that something is always working no matter how bleak things may appear. It answers the question "What is the best possible outcome from this situation?" or "How can I learn and grow from this situation?" You're more likely to give a task your best shot if you believe you can accomplish it.

  This focus is often useful when you're looking for a comeback after going off your wheat-free diet. Shifting your thought process to one that focuses on what you've learned from your relapse is essential to getting back on the wheat-free horse.

- **Address your negative beliefs and self-talk.** Encouraging positive self-talk doesn't mean ignoring your negative self-talk. Instead, acknowledge the presence of your negative beliefs, set them aside, and move forward with a more encouraging framework. This balanced approach keeps you in a more realistic mindset. For example, if your confidence is low that you can be successful with your new diet because you frequently fall off the wheat-free wagon, don't panic. Calmly acknowledge your beliefs and fears, set them aside, and then focus on more-positive approaches to your dietary choices.

Maintaining accountability

A good time to find an accountability buddy or group is when you're facing a major change, and revamping your diet to exclude wheat and other grains certainly counts. Being held accountable works best while your desire for change is high. It strengthens personal responsibility, and personal responsibility boosts motivation. Accountability characterizes your commitment and determines your level of ownership in completing the task at hand. With accountability, the impetus is on you to get it done, not on someone else doing it for you.

Ask a trusted confidant who holds your best interest at heart to be your accountability partner. Ideally, it should be someone who's ready to take the dietary plunge at the same time. You'll each be more likely to be sympathetic to each other as you experience similar challenges. If you can't find a person willing to go at the wheat-free challenge with you, consider a professional nutritionist, wellness coach, or personal fitness trainer. If you're paying your accountability partner for his professional services, not living up to your end of the bargain can get awfully expensive.

Here are a few things your partner can do to see that you stay strong with your dietary commitment:

- ✔ Act as your encourager
- ✔ Brainstorm new and different ideas with you
- ✔ Celebrate your victories with you
- ✔ Help you stay focused on your motivators and goals
- ✔ Push you to go outside of your comfort zone

Report to your accountability buddy daily or weekly with an update of your progress. You can do it by e-mail, text message, or telephone, but make sure it happens.

Discovering Your Priorities and Developing Effective Goals

The first step to identifying your priorities and creating well-written goals is to disengage from the distractions of life as we discuss earlier in the chapter. The next step is to devise a vision and a plan to help you reach it by establishing priorities and goals. Your goals are stepping stones to reaching your vision. Where do you want to be three months from now? What can you do each week to help you reach your vision?

Determining what's important to you

When you pay attention to what your body is telling you, you're better able to recognize what it needs. Needs, when left unmet, easily define what your priorities are. After you become aware of your body's needs, you can design a health vision with what's most important to you in mind. Answering the questions "What's most important to me right now?" and "Why?" is what drives you to do what you do. Whether you realize it or not, your behaviors stem from your answers to these questions. Bottom line: You're only going to do what you want to do. Unfortunately, what you want to do isn't always what you should do.

How do you increase your desire to take action when you aren't motivated? First, gather as much information as you can about the pros and cons of eliminating wheat or all grains from your diet. Then ask yourself, "What's most important to me right now?"

At first glance, it's a simple question with a simple answer, but to answer it flippantly doesn't increase motivation. When you consider the question as it relates to deep-seated emotions within you, however, you have an extremely powerful motivator that can supersede any other desire. The follow-up question "Why?" is what actually gets to the heart of your motivation

For example, most people cite good health, more energy, or weight loss as what's most important to them about going wheat-free. These same people often answer the second question — "Why?" — with emotional desires like wanting to live longer to enjoy relationships with their children and grandchildren. This emotional response is what generates the behavioral change toward eating a wheat-free, low-carb diet.

Creating a health vision

Before you begin designing your wheat-free goals, write a two- or three-sentence health vision describing what you'd look and feel like at your best. A vision is energizing and inspiring. It motivates and propels you into action. This healthy, realistic view of where you want to see yourself in the future can be an image of you six months from now or years down the road. It lays the groundwork for your three-month and weekly goals.

This health vision is your vision, not someone else's vision for you.

When writing your health vision, consider the following:

- What's most important to me? Why?
- What do I look like when I'm at my best?
- What do I feel like when I'm at my best?
- What are my motivators?
- What are my barriers?
- What are my strengths?

An example health vision may read, "I want to have enough energy as I age to play with my grandchildren and to travel with my spouse. I see myself at a constant, normal weight. I know that I'll greatly reduce my risk of developing any chronic illnesses, increase my energy level, and manage my weight by eliminating wheat from my diet." After you've written your health vision, post it in your car or on your computer, refrigerator, or bathroom mirror to remind yourself of it daily.

Writing goals to achieve your priorities

Well-written goals are the foundation of the change process and essential for long-term success. By connecting your priorities to your health vision, you map out your plan of action.

After you've completed your health vision, you're ready to set your *three-month goals*. These goals are wheat-free behaviors that you want to be performing consistently three months from now that you aren't currently acting on. They should be in direct line with and connected to your vision.

Breaking down the benefits of goal setting

The following list includes several reasons you should set goals:

- They help you understand what's most important to you.
- They provide a sense of accomplishment.
- They create purpose and meaning.
- They measure your progress.
- They hold you accountable.

- They help motivate and inspire you.
- They help to break down overwhelming aspirations into more achievable actions.
- They help increase self-confidence.
- They help organize your time.
- They give you the direction and control to change your life.

Getting SMART about your goals

We recommend following the SMART goal model when writing your goals. Some of the terms vary slightly from model to model, but for our purposes, SMART goals are

- ✔ **Specific:** This aspect answers the questions "Who? What? When? Where?" It tightens the goal and doesn't allow for any wiggle room or ambiguity.

- ✔ **Measurable:** This element answers the questions "How much? How many? How often? How do I know when I complete the goal?" When measuring the goal, your completion rate should be 60 to 80 percent. If you fall below a 60-percent success rate, the goal is probably too challenging. If you're above 80 percent with your completion rate, your goal is probably not challenging enough.

- ✔ **Action-based:** This component of the goal answers the question "What do I need to do?" You must be able to see yourself in your mind's eye performing the goal. The goal is something that you plan to do, not what you plan to not do.

- ✔ **Realistic or relevant:** This area answers the questions "Is the goal I've set realistic for me? Is the goal relevant to my vision?"

- ✔ **Timely:** This section answers the question "What is the start date and finish date of the goal?"

Brainstorming is a great way to generate ideas for your goals. Developing a list of everything that comes to mind is sure to create an a-ha moment that can propel you into action.

Weekly goals are the small steps you take toward meeting your long-term goals. They're a smaller-scale reflection of your three-month goals and health vision. The same guidelines that apply to writing three-month goals are relevant to weekly goals.

Crafting solid goals

In addition to making your goals SMART, you want to make them achievable. Unfortunately, most people set goals without actually considering whether they can execute them. Here are some tips to guide your goal-writing session:

- ✔ Remember that goals can be either mental or behavioral.

- ✔ Always start your goal with "I will."

- ✔ Make your goal a do, not a don't.

- ✔ When setting goals for your diet, set no more than two weekly goals per week and two to three three-month goals.

- ✔ Include a comment after the goal that explains the "why" of the goal.

An example of a properly written behavioral three-month goal may read as follows:

> GOAL: I will be preparing five wheat-free dinners a week at 6:00 p.m., Monday through Friday, for my family.

> COMMENT: After I totally eliminate wheat from my diet, I'll be able to help my family do the same.

An example of a properly written mental weekly goal may read

> GOAL: I will make a list of all the benefits of eliminating wheat and grains from my diet on Monday from 8:00 a.m. to 9:00 a.m.

> COMMENT: This list will help me move from the contemplation stage to the preparation stage in changing my diet.

After you finish your list of goals, rate your level of confidence that you'll complete the goal. Use a scale of one to ten, with ten being the most confident. Research indicates that those who rank their confidence at six or lower are more likely not to complete the goal. If you find yourself scoring something lower than seven, rework the goal so that your level of confidence toward it passes that threshold of seven.

Evaluating your goals

Goals don't mean much if you don't know how well you're meeting them, so you need to measure your progress every so often. At the end of each week, assess the progress of your weekly goals by asking yourself these questions:

- What went well?
- What was challenging?
- What did I learn?
- How did my success or failure feel?
- What can I do differently next week?
- What was my goal completion percentage?

Every three or four weeks, assess the progress of your three-month goals by asking yourself the weekly questions plus the following to make sure you're still connected to your long-term goals:

- Is this goal still important to me?
- What have I learned about myself in regards to this goal?

Chapter 6

Combining Wheat-Free and Other Lifestyles

*T*raditionally, the word *diet* implies food restrictions. People on "diets" change the amount and type of food they eat in order to produce weight or fat loss, create an improvement in health, or observe certain religious or ethical guidelines. But really, the word *diet* simply describes what a person eats — healthy, unhealthy, or somewhere in between. That second, broader definition is what we mean by "diet."

In this chapter, we discuss several different dietary principles that people practice, usually for perceived health purposes. Some of these restrictions support the wheat/grain-free lifestyle, whereas others may present a greater challenge in living wheat- or grain-free.

Merging Wheat-Free with Common Diets

At some point in time, most people jump on the next great dietary idea all in the name of weight loss and, to a lesser degree, good health. But are these dietary bandwagons healthy? The true test of a diet program's effectiveness is whether you can maintain the weight loss and improved health for years to come, not just for a few months.

In the following sections, we explain how eliminating wheat and grains affects other popular dietary choices. In some cases, the dual diets work well together. In other instances, adopting a particular diet is unnecessary if you're eating a wheat/grain-free diet.

Trying to eliminate fat and cholesterol

The two main issues that are falsely associated with a diet high in cholesterol and fat are obesity and heart disease. Because people want to avoid gaining weight and having heart problems, they try to cut fat and cholesterol from their diet. However, when dietary fat is decreased, by definition carbohydrates are increased. Naturally fatty foods — meat, for example — don't usually contain carbohydrates, and foods with natural carbohydrates — such as potatoes — don't contain fat. This leads to increased fat storage and heart disease.

Cutting out fat and cholesterol leads to a host of problems. First of all, ingesting cholesterol doesn't increase your blood cholesterol. Every cell in the body makes cholesterol. In fact, about 85 percent of all cholesterol is made by the body; only about 15 percent comes from food.

Second, the paradigm that cholesterol is at the root of heart disease is problematic. Statistics show that 25 percent of all heart attack victims have desirable levels of LDL-C (the "bad cholesterol"), so another mechanism is clearly at play here. And yet the thresholds for prescribing cholesterol drugs get lower and lower. The resulting higher triglycerides from eating carbohydrates such as wheat and grains are taxied around the body by LDL particles; then the LDL becomes oxidized, creating free radicals leading to inflammation. This inflammation is the beginning of heart disease, Alzheimer's disease, and other chronic illnesses. Higher cholesterol with no inflammation means no heart disease.

Therefore, this dietary restriction isn't compatible with a healthy, wheat- or grain-free diet.

Steering clear of dairy

Many people have abandoned dairy products because of their lactose and casein content.

Lactase is the enzyme that breaks down the sugar *lactose,* which is found in milk. When your body doesn't have lactase, you're considered *lactose intolerant;* you can't metabolize this sugar, so it causes gastric distress. *Casein* is a protein also present in milk. Some people react to it as an allergen, so they avoid all dairy products. Lactose intolerance and casein allergies frequently occur simultaneously in people, even though they're different conditions altogether.

One very important factor to consider when eliminating dairy from your diet is the difference between dairy-free and nondairy. A dairy-free product doesn't contain any milk and is therefore safe for those people with lactose and casein problems.

However, processed nondairy foods, such as salad dressings and nutrition bars, are allowed to contain casein and may therefore present problems for those who can't tolerate casein. Always read the label to make sure you're getting what you need.

Regardless of your need for choosing eliminating dairy, this dietary choice doesn't conflict with a wheat- or grain-free lifestyle.

Cutting out red meat

People who eliminate red meat from their diets often do so because they believe the meat's saturated fat and cholesterol content increase their chances of heart disease and cancer. However, in and of itself, red meat provides many fats and proteins essential for good health. How the meat affects your health is the result of the way the animals providing the meat are raised.

What the animal eats, you eat. Grain-fed meat creates an unhealthy ratio of omega-6 fatty acids to omega-3 fatty acids. Over time, this imbalance creates inflammation, which contributes to many diseases. Grass-fed meat, on the other hand, has a much lower (more reasonable) fatty-acid ratio. (Head to Chapter 18 for information on omega-3 and omega-6 fatty acids and ratios.)

So as long as you're purchasing grass-fed meat, you can (and should) continue to eat red meat on a wheat- or grain-free diet.

Following a lowfat, low-calorie diet

Some diets require you to significantly cut back the number of calories you consume every day. The average American needs between 2,000 and 2,600 calories, depending on gender, age, and activity level. Diets that require you to reduce the number of calories you consume often want you to cut 800 to 1,000 calories a day from your diet. Supposedly, the calorie deficit that's created pushes your body into fat-burning mode.

However, with a reduction of calories (including sugar and refined carbohydrates) comes a reduction in metabolism. A drop this significant brings your metabolism almost to a standstill, meaning your body is burning fewer calories at rest and is in a constant state of hunger. At some point, your hunger will overcome your desire to further cut your calories, which is why severe calorie restriction for weight loss and health doesn't last long-term.

The biggest challenge with low-calorie diets is overcoming the incorrect belief that the key to good health and weight loss is restricting calorie and dietary fat intake. One of the first cuts in a low-calorie diet is fat because it has nine calories per gram compared to four calories per gram for carbohydrates and proteins. But actually, your body needs fat because it's essential for the absorption of the fat-soluble vitamins A, D, E, and K. Fat also transports nutrients across cell membranes and supports cell growth. A diet high in fat "teaches" your body how to burn fat as its primary fuel source by creating ketones, a byproduct of fat metabolism. One notable ketone, beta-hydroxybutyrate, is known to be superior for brain health.

Diets that cut out fat and fat calories aren't conducive to a wheat- or grain-free lifestyle. The healthy fats in a wheat- or grain-free diet help keep you satiated; without them, your only option is to try to fill up on wheat and other carbs, which keeps the gnawing hunger at bay only in the short term.

On some reduced-calorie diets, after you hit your goal weight you're allowed to gradually reintroduce foods you'd stopped eating while you were trying to lose weight. However, this reintroduction strategy doesn't apply to the wheat, grains, and sugar you've cut from your diet. Eliminating wheat, grains, and added sugars is a permanent change.

Pairing Paleo with Wheat-Free

Paleo has its foundation rooted in man's diet during the Paleolithic era. It's sometimes called the caveman diet because it's based on the hunter-gatherers' diet of meats, fruits, and vegetables. Interestingly, the human genetic makeup is virtually the same as it was during the Paleolithic era. (Grains weren't introduced until later, in the Neolithic era.)

Paleo's anti-inflammatory approach helps stabilize blood sugar, insulin, and leptin and eliminates leaky gut through a grain-free, low-carbohydrate diet high in healthy fats. (Chapter 4 has details on how eating grains affects blood sugar, insulin, and leptin.)

The dietary principles of a Paleo lifestyle align pretty closely with those of a wheat/grain-free lifestyle. You eat simple foods and avoid processed ones. For example, Paleo-friendly proteins should be grass-fed, organic, or wild-caught. As for oils, you can use almond oil, coconut oil, olive oil, and palm oil, among others. Organic veggies are a staple of the Paleo lifestyle.

When it comes to fruits, you have to be cautious. Today's fruit is nothing like the fruit of the Paleolithic era. Today, it's available 12 months out of the year, which isn't natural; your caveman ancestors ate only the fruit that was in season. Today's fruit is also much larger and sweeter; that makes it easy to overeat, which can cause blood sugar spikes and insulin reactions. Therefore, Paleo recommends focusing your produce intake on veggies over fruits.

The fruits you do eat should be organic, and those with low levels of fructose are best for regular consumption. Try apples, blueberries, cherries, raspberries, strawberries, tangerines, and blackberries.

A Paleo lifestyle goes a bit farther than wheat-free living in terms of what you cut out of your diet. Going Paleo requires that you give up grains, beans and legumes, dairy, white potatoes, seed oils, anything with added sugar, anything processed, and most alcoholic beverages.

Within the Paleo community, several foods are controversial topics. For instance, some devotees consume tubers and maple syrup, and others don't. Understanding how your body reacts to certain carbohydrates is key in determining what foods you can tolerate.

To supplement a healthy eating plan, you also follow some simple rules when living Paleo that are meant to help you feel better mentally and physically:

✔ Get adequate amounts of quality sleep.

✔ Participate in physical activity in the form of play and exercise.

✔ Practice positive self-talk.

✔ Follow stress-management techniques regularly.

If, after reading this section, you want more information about the Paleo lifestyle, check out *Living Paleo For Dummies* by Melissa Joulwan and Dr. Kellyann Petrucci (Wiley).

Living Vegetarian and Wheat-Free

At first glance, it may seem contradictory to mention a wheat/grain-free, low-carb lifestyle and vegetarianism in the same sentence. Vegetarianism is all about carbs, particularly when you stick primarily to fruits, vegetables, and grains. Many people expand their diets by drinking soft drinks and eating chips, all in the name of vegetarianism.

Maintaining a vegetarian diet while eliminating wheat, added sugar, and vegetable and seed oils would be quite a challenge because of the blood sugar–raising effects of many fruits. Reducing the amount of fructose necessary to keep blood sugar levels down means cutting back on several types of fruits such as watermelon, raisins, and bananas.

Our DNA was never designed to handle vegetarianism, especially when you have to take supplements, such as vitamin B-12, to meet your nutritional needs. Additionally, reducing cholesterol levels with a lowfat diet causes vitamin D deficiencies (vitamin D is synthesized via cholesterol).

The most basic definition of vegetarianism is that vegetarians don't eat meat. However, many variations of vegetarianism exist. Here's a look at a few sub-categories of vegetarianism and how they do or don't relate to a wheat/grain-free lifestyle.

- **Fruitarianism:** *Fruitarianism* can be defined in several different ways, but generally speaking, fruitarians eat only or mostly fruit; stricter adherents avoid nuts, seeds, and grains — anything that can be harvested. True, a fruitarian diet is usually grain-free, but it's far from ideal. The stress it places on the liver (from an excess of fructose, an omega-6 fatty acid overload if nuts are included, and a lack of dietary fat) greatly jeopardizes your health. Therefore, we don't recommend fruitarianism, even though its grain restrictions involve eliminating wheat.

- **Lacto-ovo vegetarian:** Lacto-ovo vegetarians eliminate all meat, but do eat eggs and dairy products. (*Lacto* is Latin for "milk," and *ovo* is Latin for "egg.") This allows great latitude for vegetarians. Eliminating wheat and other grains from a lacto-ovo vegetarian diet is possible, but the high carbohydrate content that still remains will elevate blood sugar and triglyceride levels. Keeping fat in the diet by eating eggs and dairy will help in raising HDL (good cholesterol) numbers.

- **Pescatarian:** Although not considered true vegetarians, *pescatarians* eat fish and seafood with their otherwise-vegetarian diet. Typically, most people have elevated omega-6 fatty acid levels. When combined with low levels of omega-3 fatty acids, inflammation occurs and disease results. Because fish are rich in omega-3 fatty acids, pescatarianism may help balance omega-6 and omega-3 fatty acids. By sticking to a pescatarian diet that's also free from wheat, grains, and vegetable oil, this high ratio can be reduced to the desirable 1:1.

- **Raw food:** Though a raw diet doesn't expressly forbid eating meat, it does shun cooking food at temperatures higher than 118 degrees. Therefore, most raw food folks are vegetarians. The theory is that cooking the food any hotter saps the enzymes necessary for proper digestion. The problem with this idea is that the body, not the food itself, provides all the enzymes needed for digestion. By eliminating wheat and grains from a raw food diet, a diet similar to pescatarianism may emerge.

- **Veganism:** *Veganism* is a lifestyle that promotes respect to all animals. In the truest sense, vegans steer clear of all products that exploit animals. That means not only avoiding eating meat, dairy, eggs, and so on but also refusing to wear fur and leather or use products tested on animals. Vegans eat all fruits, vegetables, grains, beans, and legumes. Veganism is deficient in certain vitamins and minerals and deficient in fat to the point of producing unhealthy cholesterol numbers and elevated blood sugar levels, which is why we don't recommend pairing this form of vegetarianism with a wheat- or grain-free lifestyle.

A vegetarian diet isn't synonymous with a healthy diet. A person who only eats potato chips and cookies and drinks soda would be considered a vegetarian but far from healthy.

Navigating Other Dietary Philosophies

The following philosophies and diets aren't followed as widely as the diets we talk about earlier in the chapter. However, you may already follow one of the plans listed here, so we include them to give you an idea of how a wheat/grain-free lifestyle can work with these specific diets.

Many of these programs have some validity because they reduce or eliminate the sugar and refined carbohydrates that are responsible for weight gain and a major player in chronic illnesses. However, some of these philosophies and diets need a major facelift to meet the high expectations of a wheat/grain-free, low-carb, no-vegetable-oil diet. We've given a brief description of each practice and noted whether it's conducive to maintaining good health and weight loss as part of your wheat/grain-free lifestyle:

- ✔ **Gluten-free:** Eliminating gluten from your diet means one of two things: You're eating a naturally gluten-free diet of meats, fruits, and vegetables or you're eating commercial gluten-free foods that have had the gluten removed and starch added (see Chapter 3 for more in-depth information on wheat and gluten). The added starch in the latter causes the pancreas to secrete insulin, which escorts the glucose (starch) to fat cells to be stored for later use. Therefore, naturally restricting gluten by eliminating wheat and grains is the way to go.

- ✔ **Hormone- and antibiotic-free:** Many manufacturers pump animals full of hormones and antibiotics to help beef up the animals (pun intended) before they're slaughtered and to treat the illnesses they pick up in their poor living conditions. Eating products from such animals means you're consuming larger amounts of omega-6 fatty acids. That's why we recommend following this dietary restriction as part of your wheat/grain-free lifestyle.

Taking a stand against consuming hormone- and antibiotic-treated products also supports humane animal treatment. Cows and chickens are much happier and healthier when raised in their natural surroundings — grazing in a pasture with space to move about and ingesting grass, not corn feed.

✔ **Anti-inflammatory:** Inflammation can strike anywhere in the body, from joints and muscles to various tissues. Research shows that what you eat influences the level of inflammation in your body, with wheat, sugar, and many plant and seed oils being the biggest culprits. Eliminating these items greatly reduces inflammation and helps restore the body — and matches very closely to our wheat/grain-free recommendations — so we support incorporating anti-inflammatory principles into your new lifestyle.

✔ **Kosher:** *Kosher* foods are those that meet the strict guidelines of the Jewish dietary law. A kosher diet places restrictions on what kinds of meat, seafood, and dairy you can eat and on eating meat and dairy together. But plenty of foods exist that allow you to maintain a wheat/grain-free kosher diet, so this philosophy is a viable way of living wheat/grain-free.

✔ **Organic:** Foods that are raised *organically* don't use pesticides, chemical fertilizers, genetic modification, irradiation, sewage sludge, growth hormones, or antibiotics. This approach ensures healthier living conditions throughout the plant or animal's life. We strongly recommend eating organic as a way of bettering your health. You can do so with little bearing on your wheat/grain-free diet (you just have to be more watchful of whether your meat, produce, and so on is organic).

✔ **Sugar-free:** Eliminating carbohydrates that are the easiest to digest, such as table sugar, pasta, potatoes, and bread, are at the heart of a *sugar-free diet.* After this, the debate begins. Your level of sugar sensitivity to fruit, sweet potatoes, dairy products, and any other carbohydrate-rich food dictates the degree to which you can eat these items. Part of going wheat/grain-free is eliminating added sugars from your diet, so this philosophy definitely fits with a wheat/grain-free lifestyle.

✔ **Supplement or the latest food trend:** You've probably known someone who raved about going on the cabbage soup diet, the grapefruit diet, or some other similar weight-loss plan. The idea that a single supplement or food is the panacea of good health is short-sighted, to say the least. No one item leads to optimal health; in fact, hanging your hat on one food to meet all your nutritional needs can be extremely dangerous. Not only does doing so deny your body important nutrients, but it also creates a situation where you never learn how to eat intelligently. Therefore, we don't recommend this philosophy period; it has no place in a wheat/grain-free lifestyle.

Chapter 7

Stocking a Wheat-Free Kitchen

*I*f you've been eating like the average American eats, you likely have shelves filled with foods that contain wheat. Those have to go if you're going to succeed at living wheat-free. Deciphering food labels is most of the battle when it comes to stocking the shelves at home and finding your way through the endless options at the grocery store. In this chapter, we steer you to the most important parts of the label with regards to wheat-free living and show you wheat's and sugar's various disguises. Eating the right foods helps you rid yourself of cravings and low blood sugar, as well as the subtle pains in your joints and stomach.

We also walk you through the process of emptying your pantry and refrigerator of items containing wheat and restocking with good-for-you wheat-free items. This shift requires you to clear out space in the fridge because you find yourself increasingly buying fresh foods rather than packaged products that can sit in your pantry for years and years.

Reviewing Food Labels in the Spirit of a Wheat-Free Lifestyle

Understanding food labels is paramount to living a healthy wheat-free life. The basic info that the law requires every food item to post is your guide to keeping or tossing a food item. Food labels contain two categories of information:

> ✔ The nutrition facts section lists the actual grams of fat, carbs, and protein as well as cholesterol, sodium, fiber, sugar, and various vitamins and minerals. Calorie count tops the list.

✔ The ingredients list spells out the components that make up the food, beginning with the most prevalent ingredient. Sometimes this list can be so confusing — with various difficult-to-pronounce names — you'd think you were in a chemistry class. (Those foods are usually the processed ones you should shy away from.)

Most people just avoid looking at food labels altogether and grab a box of whatever, thinking ignorance is bliss. However, you'll soon be able to make quick work of these labels. In the following sections, we explain how the nutrition details apply to wheat-free eating, and we give you a quick guide to ferreting out wheat on food labels.

Being in-the-know about nutrition facts

The nutrition facts label exists to simplify your understanding of what a food contains, although its setup is sometimes more confusing than helpful. For our purposes, you need to focus mostly on the listings in the following sections.

Contrary to popular practice, we aren't going to focus on calories. Not that calories don't count in some capacity, but when you rid your diet of wheat and added sugar, your food intake tends to self-regulate. Counting calories won't be an issue.

The other info we don't cover is the protein content. Cutting out wheat doesn't mean blowing up your protein intake like many critics suggest. Actually, most wheat-free diets have a similar protein content that the body seems to regulate very well.

Serving size

Don't confuse serving size with how much you can eat in one sitting. A serving size isn't about how much you feel like eating. You must read what the manufacturer considers to be a serving because that amount is what the nutrition facts are calculated on. If the box says a serving of mac and cheese is ½ cup and you eat 1½ cups, you've really consumed three times the amount of calories, fat, and so on listed in the nutrition facts. Big difference! A quick way to estimate the serving size without busting out a measuring cup is to read the "servings per container" number, which is always located near the serving size.

Checking the label is especially important because not all foods in the same category necessarily have the same recommended serving size. In the case of cereals, you often see quite a difference among serving sizes depending on the density of the product. For example, a serving of Cereal A is ½ cup, while Cereal B is 1 cup. (Of course, both cereal and mac and cheese contain wheat, so they don't have a place in your pantry anyway. We're just using these examples to illustrate the concept of serving size.) But serving size is still important even for healthy foods such as fruits. One type of frozen berry may have a ¾-cup serving, while another may list ½ cup. You want to know how many servings of fruit you're really taking in so you can minimize the potential blood sugar spike.

Trans fats

What were once the darlings of the food industry are now the bane of health practitioners. Laboratory-made *trans fats* lead to a longer shelf life for the product, but they don't do the same for your body. Trans fats raise your LDL (bad) cholesterol and lower your HDL (good) cholesterol.

You should avoid these fats completely because they're associated with an increased risk for heart disease, breast cancer, obesity, diabetes, depression, asthma, and osteoporosis. Commercial baked goods such as cakes, cookies, and crackers have trans fats. So do fried foods such as doughnuts and French fries, as well as most shortenings and margarines. Thankfully, the food industry has felt the pressure from government and the medical community and begun removing trans fats from some foods.

Don't be fooled by the label, however. Companies are allowed to list trans fat content at 0 grams as long as the product contains less than 0.5 grams. So 0 doesn't necessarily mean 0. Half a gram may not sound like a lot, but eat a few servings and your trans fats intake becomes more substantial. Even if a label lists 0 grams of trans fat, look for the words "hydrogenated" or "partially hydrogenated" to spot hidden amounts.

Cholesterol

Many people check the cholesterol content of a food because they're concerned a high number will raise their blood cholesterol, but you can pretty much ignore this part of the label. Eating cholesterol doesn't actually increase your measured cholesterol levels. Your body produces about 85 percent of its cholesterol on its own; even if you ingest 0 milligrams of the substance, your body will still produce cholesterol. As the body tends to do, it will lower its production of cholesterol if you eat too much and raise its production if you don't ingest enough. So don't fret about this number.

That doesn't mean that your diet doesn't affect your cholesterol levels. Wheat is a carbohydrate, and other carbs do raise your cholesterol. The chain reaction that follows the elevated blood glucose eventually leads to higher LDL levels and inflammation.

Remember: All that being said, if your doctor has put you on a low-cholesterol diet for medical reasons, we don't advocate going off that diet without first consulting him.

Total carbohydrates

Fiber and sugar are categorized as carbohydrates on nutrition labels. However, they each get their own line of information so you can see how much of each one the food contains.

✔ **Fiber:** Fiber is beneficial in reducing your insulin response and helping move the food along the digestive tract. However, not all fiber is created equal. The fiber you want comes from fruits and veggies, not wheat and other so-called healthy whole grains. In fact, eating fresh foods such as spinach, Swiss chard, asparagus, blackberries, and raspberries provides as much or more fiber than snack foods fortified with fiber.

   Most people don't get enough fiber on a daily basis. Shoot for about 25 grams for women and 40 grams for men. The reality, however, is that you shouldn't need to keep track of fiber if you're on a wheat-free lifestyle. You'll get plenty.

✔ **Sugar:** The sugar category needs extra attention because sugar can cause blood sugar to rise just as much as wheat and other grains can. Both sugar and wheat cause inflammation, and both trigger cravings to eat more; these cravings lead to fat storage, heart disease, and diabetes. Eat the lowest-sugar foods you can. (Because you can't tell from the nutrition facts where the sugar content in a food comes from, you have to dig deeper in the ingredients list; check out the later "Recognizing sugar's many pseudonyms" section for more on this task.)

Scrutinizing the ingredients list

If a food product has "wheat" in the name — for example, wheat crackers — you can be pretty certain the item contains wheat. (One exception: buckwheat, which isn't wheat or even a grain at all.) Otherwise, you have to read the ingredients list to know for sure whether a food contains wheat.

Your first stop should be the bottom of the ingredients list. By law, any item that contains one of eight major food allergens (including wheat) must specifically say so. The sample label in Figure 7-1 spells it out in bold print: contains wheat, milk, and soy ingredients.

At this point, all you know is that the food contains wheat. Normally, that's all you need to know, but perhaps you've already eaten something and now want to check the label (or you're giving yourself a little wheat-eating leeway for a special occasion, as we discuss in Chapter 15.) To find out how prominent wheat ingredients are in an item, head back to the top of the ingredients list and start scanning. The closer the ingredient is to the beginning of the list, the more of that ingredient the food contains.

You also have to read the lists within the list. Some food items are made up of ingredients that have their own ingredients. Check out Figure 7-1, which shows an ingredient list for cereal bars. The cereal has its own list of ingredients (shown in parentheses), which are required to be listed on the label of the final product. The cereal contains three forms of wheat: whole grain wheat, wheat bran, and soluble wheat fiber. If you skip over these subingredients, you may miss a wheat listing (or three).

Figure 7-1:
Wheat is listed multiple times in the ingredients list for cereal bars.

Nutrition Facts

Serving Size 1 Bar (22g)

Amount Per Serving

Calories 90	Calories from Fat 15

	% Daily Value*
Total Fat 2g	3%
Saturated Fat 1g	5%
Trans Fat 0g	
Cholesterol 0mg	0%
Sodium 90mg	4%
Total Carbohydrate 17g	6%
Dietary Fiber 3g	10%
Sugars 6g	
Protein less than 1g	

Vitamin A	0%	•	Vitamin C	0%
Calcium	0%	•	Iron	0%
Thiamin	10%	•	Riboflavin	10%
Niacin	10%	•	Vitamin B$_6$	10%

Percent Daily Values are based on a 2,000 calorie diet. Your daily values may be higher or lower depending on your calorie needs.

	Calorie	2,000	2,500
Total Fat	Less than	65g	80g
Saturated Fat	Less than	20g	25g
Cholesterol	Less than	300mg	300mg
Sodium	Less than	2,400mg	2,400mg
Total Carbohydrate		300g	375g
Dietary Fiber		25g	30g

INGREDIENTS: CEREAL (RICE, WHOLE GRAIN WHEAT, SUGAR, WHEAT BRAN, SOLUBLE WHEAT FIBER, SALT, MALT FLAVORING, MALTODEXTRIN, THIAMIN MONONITRATE [VITAMIN B$_1$], RIBOFLAVIN [VITAMIN B$_2$]), SOLUBLE CORN FIBER, FRUCTOSE, CORN SYRUP, SUGAR, VEGETABLE OIL (PARTIALLY HYDROGENATED PALM KERNEL AND SOYBEAN OIL, SOYBEAN AND PALM OIL WITH TBHQ FOR FRESHNESS) †, MALTODEXTRIN, CONTAINS TWO PERCENT OR LESS OF WHOLE GRAIN OATS, DEXTROSE, WHEAT FLOUR, SORBITOL, GLYCERIN, BROWN SUGAR (SUGAR, MOLASSES), APPLESAUCE (APPLES, WATER), NATURAL AND ARTIFICIAL VANILLA FLAVOR, NONFAT DRY MILK, SOY LECITHIN, NATURAL AND ARTIFICIAL FLAVOR, SALT, COLOR ADDED, NIACINAMIDE, PYRIDOXINE HYDROCHLORIDE (VITAMIN B$_6$), BHT (PRESERVATIVE).
† LESS THAN 0.5g TRANS FAT PER SERVING.

CONTAINS WHEAT, MILK AND SOY INGREDIENTS.

© John Wiley & Sons, Inc.

Not all wheat ingredients conveniently contain the word *wheat* in the name. Check out the following section for problematic ingredients you may not think to watch for.

Picking out wheat by any other name

As you become better at identifying which foods contain wheat, your ability to make better food choices improves. When you read an ingredients list, the easiest word to look for is *wheat*, but you should also be on the lookout for these other words:

- Barley grass (because of cross-contamination)
- Bulgur (a form of wheat)
- Durum, durum flour, durum wheat
- Einkorn
- Emmer
- Farina
- Flour (including all-purpose, cake, enriched, graham, high-protein or high-gluten, and pastry)
- Farro
- Fu
- Kamut
- Seitan (made from wheat gluten and commonly used in vegetarian meals)
- Semolina
- Spelt
- Sprouted wheat
- Triticale (a cross between wheat and rye)
- Triticum aestivum
- Wheat berries
- Wheat bran, germ/germ oil/germ extract, gluten, grass, malt, or starch
- Wheat protein/hydrolyzed wheat protein

Recognizing sugar's many pseudonyms

Food companies are allowed to separate the various types of sugars in the ingredients list with different names, so you need to know all the different sugar aliases to truly gauge how much sugar you're eating. Because ingredients are listed from highest percentage to lowest percentage, breaking up the sugar listings can make a food seem like it has less sugar than it really does. If food manufacturers had to combine all the sugars into one listing, many foods would have to list sugar first.

Just like wheat, sugar has many different names:

- Agave nectar
- Brown sugar
- Cane crystals
- Cane sugar
- Corn sweetener
- Corn syrup
- Crystalline fructose
- Dextrose
- Evaporated cane juice
- Fructose
- Fruit juice concentrates
- Glucose
- High fructose corn syrup
- Honey
- Invert sugar
- Lactose
- Maltose
- Malt syrup
- Molasses
- Raw sugar
- Sucrose
- Sugar
- Syrup

Cleaning Out the Kitchen

For some people, wrapping their brains around throwing away unspoiled food may be the first obstacle to overcome. Some habits are difficult to break, but realize that tossing every box of cereal, can of soup, and package of frozen waffles is saving you from gas and bloating today and heart disease and diabetes down the road. Your blood pressure may be rising a bit now thinking about all the stuff you have to chuck, but you're doing it a favor in the long run.

The best way to determine which foods should stay and which foods should go is to read the ingredients lists on the food labels. Reading every label may seem daunting, but you'll quickly get the hang of spotting the usual suspects. (The earlier section "Scrutinizing the ingredients list" helps you suss out these offenders.) And practicing with the items your own kitchen prepares you for reading labels when you go to the grocery store to restock your kitchen with wheat-free foods.

Toss any perishable items in the trash. Even leftovers from last night need to go. The time to change is now. Donate all unopened, nonperishable packages to a food bank.

In a perfect world, everyone in your household would be going along with your new wheat-free plan. That ideal isn't always the case, however. If you do share the kitchen with these eaters, designate certain shelves and drawers for your wheat-free foods. You're just trying to limit temptation. And don't give up on that perfect world. As others see your health and energy levels improve, they may be motivated to make the same dietary changes. Voilà! Wheat-free household.

Going through the cabinets and pantry

The pantry is probably the biggest culprit in most kitchens. Think about all the food you store in there that likely contains wheat. Here's a list to get you started:

- ✔ Bread
- ✔ Cakes and cookies
- ✔ Doughnuts
- ✔ Pasta

✔ Cereal

✔ Flour

✔ Chips

✔ Certain alcoholic drinks (if you're giving up wheat because of a problem with gluten; see Chapter 15 for a breakdown of what isn't wheat-free)

✔ Canned soups

✔ Crackers

Everything on this list has to go. And as you sort through items one by one, you'll probably find more foods that violate the wheat-free plan. Toss 'em all!

Getting these items out of your sight is essential because temptation can make you crazy. Throwing out tons of items you spent good money on may seem daunting, but replacing them with foods that truly nourish your body can be invigorating.

The following list provides a few more items that, although they don't actually contain wheat, are important to omit in the context of better health and feeling good. For starters, monosodium glutamate (MSG) is a very common food additive that causes many of the same side effects as wheat (in addition to having its own addictive properties). Another category of food to toss is common vegetable-based cooking oils. Although some oils have been touted as healthy alternatives to animal fats, they can be far from it. They contain high ratios of omega-6 to omega-3 fatty acids and are highly processed. Along with wheat and grains, high ratios of omega-6 to omega-3 are associated with an increase in all inflammatory diseases. These oils appear in most boxed foods, and you may have bottles of them for cooking or baking.

✔ Seed cooking oils (canola, corn, vegetable, soybean, and sunflower, just to name a few)

✔ Foods with added sugars

✔ Foods containing MSG

✔ Foods containing hydrogenated or partially hydrogenated oils

✔ Foods containing trans fats

The focus of a wheat-free diet is, of course, eliminating wheat. But many grains cause some of the same effects as wheat in many people, so we also support ridding your kitchen of grain products in general as a step toward improved health.

Tossing items from the fridge and freezer

Refrigerated and frozen prepared items most likely have ingredients from the wheat and sugar lists we provide earlier in the chapter. Read the labels and be prepared to toss. Keep your eye on the prize: a great quality of life. Here are other items to be on the lookout for:

✓ Breaded meat, fish, or chicken

✓ Jellies and jams with added sugar

✓ Margarine and other "buttery" spreads

✓ Creamy salad dressings with added sugar

✓ Frozen waffles, pancakes, biscuits, or other breakfast pastries

✓ Ice cream

✓ Frozen dinners

✓ Ketchup (mostly sugar)

✓ Beer (if you're avoiding gluten)

Navigating the Grocery Store

With a knowledge of what ingredients shouldn't be heading into your body, you're ready to focus on ones that should. The grocery store becomes a more manageable proposition when you're wheat-free because the cereal, snack food, condiment, and bread aisles are nary worth a visit. Suddenly you find yourself spending most of your time shopping the perimeter of the store, where the fresh produce, meats, and dairy reside, and venturing into the middle only occasionally for staples. Natural grocery stores are a bit more expensive, but they have more wheat-free options in the prepackaged food areas (though those options may still contain vegetable oils and/or added sugar).

Don't go to the grocery store hungry, and don't venture down the snack food aisle for old times' sake. Just like Columbus went looking for Asia and ended up in the Bahamas, you may find yourself headed for the broccoli but end up buying cookies instead. In time, the temptation to visit your old wheat-filled friends will be gone. For now, eat before you go and stick to the aisles with things on your list.

In the following sections, we explain what items you should be shopping for on your wheat-free diet.

Selecting the right fruits and veggies

All fruits and vegetables are wheat-free, so you can eat most of these with abandon. Frozen, canned, and fresh are all viable options, but organic is the best option for optimum health. Frozen vegetables are sometimes even more nutritious than canned or fresh vegetables because they're frozen fresh to lock in the nutrients (whereas that wilted "fresh" kale may be on its last leg). Focus on the following types of vegetables:

- ✔ Dark, leafy greens such as spinach, kale, and collard and mustard greens
- ✔ Brightly colored vegetables such as peppers, carrots, and eggplant
- ✔ Root vegetables such as sweet potatoes, radishes, and beets
- ✔ Cruciferous vegetables such as broccoli, cabbage, cauliflower, bok choy, and Brussels sprouts
- ✔ Onions, cucumbers, celery, and mushrooms (okay, mushrooms are technically a fungus)

Limit your intake of corn and white potatoes; they aren't very nutrient-dense and cause an increase in blood sugar you don't see with other veggies. They're okay on occasion but not as a staple.

As you get used to wheat-free living with an emphasis on eating low-sugar items, you notice your tastes changing. Suddenly, the naturally occurring sugar in fruit more than satisfies your sweet cravings. But that doesn't mean you can chow down on fruit 24/7. Fruit doesn't contain wheat, of course, but even natural sugars can negatively affect your blood sugar if you eat them in large quantities. The easiest way to determine which fruits have the lowest effect on blood sugar is to categorize them by their glycemic load. This measurement tells you the impact a specific serving size of a food has on blood sugar; the lower the number, the better. Here's how some fruits compare:

- ✔ Low glycemic load: Blueberries, strawberries, raspberries, cherries, oranges, peaches, grapefruit, and watermelon.
- ✔ Medium glycemic load: Prunes and grapes.
- ✔ Medium to high glycemic load: Bananas, dates, and raisins.

Fruit juices fall into the high glycemic category because their sugars are concentrated. We recommend avoiding fruit juice altogether.

Opting for the smartest meats and seafood

Stay with the unadulterated versions of meat, chicken, and seafood. Grocery stores carry lots of seasoned and marinated prepackaged meats that inevitably contain wheat, sugar, and/or vegetable oils. Buy the raw stuff and create your own recipes. (Check out Part III for ideas.) Even better, buy grass-fed meats to take advantage of their higher amounts of anti-inflammatory omega-3 fatty acids. Great protein options include

- ✔ Red meat such as beef, bison, elk, goat, and venison.
- ✔ Poultry such as chicken, duck, and turkey.
- ✔ Pork such as loins, chops, and ribs and cured cuts such as bacon and sausage.
- ✔ Seafood, including all fish and shellfish. Canned sardines, herring, salmon, and tuna are also excellent options. The best choices are those canned in olive oil or a tomato, chili, or mustard sauce. Avoid those packed in soybean or sunflower oil.

Digging for dairy products

The dairy section can be hit or miss when it comes to acceptable wheat-free foods. Like everything else you buy, read the labels. Something as simple as yogurt can have wheat in the form of starches or mix-ins like granola or cookies. Milk can cause a blood sugar spike for some; choose higher-fat milk products to slow digestion and any blood sugar increases.

Stock your fridge with these items:

- ✔ Butter (real butter, not any type of substitute)
- ✔ Eggs (preferably pastured because of the higher omega-3 levels)
- ✔ High-fat cheese and cottage cheese
- ✔ Plain yogurt (preferably Greek because of its higher protein and lower sugar contents)
- ✔ Sour cream
- ✔ Whole milk (preferably from grass-fed cows)

Avoid most of the mass-produced brands of yogurt (particularly flavored yogurts) because they use added sugar, often in the form of high fructose corn syrup.

Choosing nuts, seeds, and oils

Nuts and seeds are a fantastic snack because they contain an assortment of nutrients; eat them raw, sprouted, or dry roasted. Nut butters are also a great option. When you're ready to grab a handful of nuts or seeds to snack on, reach for these:

- ✔ Almonds, Brazil nuts, cashews, macadamia nuts, pecans, pine nuts, and walnuts

- ✔ Chia, flax, pumpkin, sesame, and sunflower seeds

Wondering why peanuts aren't on this list? Peanuts are actually legumes. They have very high omega-6 fatty acid levels with practically no omega-3 fatty acids. Definitely a food to avoid.

Choose your oils based on how you plan to use them. If you'll cook with it, be aware of its *smoke point* (how hot it can get before breaking down). We talk about smoke points in more detail in Chapter 9, but you can use the following list as a quick guide:

- ✔ **High heat:** Almond oil, avocado oil, ghee (clarified butter)

- ✔ **Semi-high heat:** Butter, coconut oil, macadamia nut oil

- ✔ **Low heat:** Olive oil

Seed oils (such as canola oil) have no place in your healthy diet, as we explain in the earlier section "Going through the cabinets and pantry."

Part III
Easy Wheat-Free Cooking

Five Wheat- or Grain-Free Snacks to Keep on Hand

- ✔ Hard-boiled eggs
- ✔ Mixed berries
- ✔ Homemade granola (nuts, seeds, shaved unsweetened coconut)
- ✔ Avocados
- ✔ Squares of dark chocolate

Head to www.dummies.com/extras/livingwheatfree for a list of food substitutions you can try in place of off-limit items like spaghetti and buns.

In this part...

- Jump-start your day with simple wheat- and grain-free breakfast recipes that are sure to satisfy.

- Serve up a dinner entree so tasty that even the pickiest eater won't miss the wheat.

- Cut the clean-up with one-pot wonders.

- Make veggies a go-to part of every meal with a variety of side dish options.

- Whip up some indulgent snack and appetizer recipes to replace typical, unhealthy party food.

- Satisfy your sweet tooth (without sacrificing your wheat/grain-free goals) with baked goods that get their flavor from ingredients other than sugar.

Chapter 8

Starting Out Right: Breakfast

In This Chapter

▶ Moving beyond breakfast cereals for a nutritious start to the day

▶ Creating easy wheat-free breakfast dishes

We're not sure how it came to be, but a typical breakfast in the United States is a wheat feast, usually accompanied by lots and lots of sugar. How a piece of whole-wheat toast with jelly, or a bowl of sugary cereal, and a glass of fruit juice passes for a great way to start the day is beyond us.

Both of these scenarios send your blood sugar through the roof; they get you charging out the door only to have your energy plummet two or three hours later. Suddenly, the only options are the donuts on the break room table at work, which send you through the same yo-yo energy cycle.

In this chapter, we show you plenty of tasty wheat-free options to choose from at breakfast. We realize that most people are frantic in the morning trying to get themselves and the kids out the door, so we give you some quick smoothie options. On days when you have a bit more time, you can make the crepes, sausage, or casserole and then enjoy the leftovers on a busy weekday morning. Healthy and speedy; you can't beat that.

Avoiding Wheat at a Typically Wheat-Heavy Meal

If you can set your alarm clock about 10 minutes earlier in the morning, you should have enough time to make some really tasty, healthy breakfasts that the whole family will enjoy. The little ones may complain for a few days about not getting their sugar fix through cereals or pastries, but they'll soon get used to it. They'll also probably notice that their energy levels stay elevated, making paying attention in school much easier.

You have many choices for breakfast foods beyond the quick-and-easy cereal and donuts. Eggs are an excellent choice for the first meal of the day. Eggs, especially the yolks, have gotten a bad rap for the last 40 years. Doctors and dieticians across America told patients to cut the eggs from their diets because of the high cholesterol and fat content. But research now shows that ingesting cholesterol doesn't make your cholesterol go up and that the egg yolk is even more nutrient-dense than the white.

In fact, the egg yolk contains more than 90 percent of the recommended daily allowance for 14 nutrients. It even includes 100 percent of vitamins A, D, E, and K. This superfood practically replaces the need for a vitamin pill. And though most people think the white supplies all the protein, the yolk actually contains over 40 percent of the protein content in an egg. If possible, always try to get pastured eggs, which contain higher levels of omega-3 fatty acids.

We offer omelet and casserole recipes later in the chapter, but you can also serve eggs prepared other ways — fried, hard-boiled, poached, scrambled, and over-easy, among others. With all the different cooking methods, you can serve a new egg every day of the week. So much for a boring breakfast!

The Homemade Breakfast Sausage recipe in this chapter is perfect for keeping on hand in the fridge or freezer on the days when you hit the snooze button. It requires you to spend a bit of time in the kitchen, so you may want to prepare it on a weekend morning (or the night before) and serve the leftovers on mornings when time is at a premium.

Smoothies offer a chance to be creative with added flavors or nutrients. Throw in some coconut oil for a healthy fat or any type of dark green leafy vegetable to add some nutrient density.

Don't be afraid to venture out of the customary breakfast choices. Leftovers from the night before may be the easiest option and probably only require the microwave.

Easy Cream Cheese Crepes

Prep time: 4 min • **Cook time:** 15 min • **Yield:** About eight 6-inch pancakes

Ingredients	Directions
4 ounces cream cheese at room temperature **4 eggs**	*1* Blend the first three ingredients in a blender. The batter may be a bit lumpy. Let the mixture rest 2 minutes so the bubbles can settle.
4 teaspoons vanilla whey protein **Butter for greasing**	*2* Pour ⅛ of the batter into a hot skillet greased with butter. Cook for 2 minutes until golden, flip, and cook 1 minute on the other side. Repeat with the rest of the batter.

Per serving: Calories 106 (From Fat 72); Fat 8g (Saturated 4g); Cholesterol 119mg; Sodium 94mg; Carbohydrate 1g (Dietary Fiber 0g); Protein 7g.

Tip: Serve with fresh berries.

Tip: If you've never cooked crepes, see Figure 8-1 for help.

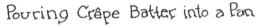

Pouring Crêpe Batter into a Pan

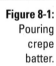

Figure 8-1: Pouring crepe batter.

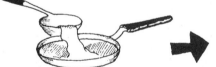

Pour the batter into the crêpe pan with a ladle or measuring cup.

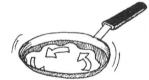

Swirl the pan around so the batter runs to the edges and covers the bottom of the pan.

Illustration by Elizabeth Kurtzman

Homemade Breakfast Sausage

Prep time: 20 min • **Cook time:** 15–20 min • **Yield:** 8 servings

Ingredients	Directions
1 pound full-fat ground pork	*1* Combine the pork, garlic, syrup, sage, thyme, salt, pepper, and cayenne in a large bowl. Gently mix with your hands until well combined. Form the mixture into sixteen 2½-inch patties about ¼ inch thick.
1 clove garlic, minced	
1½ tablespoons maple syrup	
1 teaspoon dried sage	*2* Cook half the patties in a large nonstick skillet over medium heat until well browned and cooked through, 3 to 5 minutes per side.
¼ teaspoon dried thyme	
1 teaspoon salt	
¾ teaspoon pepper	*3* Transfer to a paper towel-lined plate and cover with foil. Wipe out the skillet and repeat with the remaining patties.
⅛ teaspoon cayenne pepper	

Per serving: Calories 183 (From Fat 144); Fat 16g (Saturated 5g); Cholesterol 43mg; Sodium 330mg; Carbohydrate 2g (Dietary Fiber 0g); Protein 8g.

Note: You can refrigerate the raw sausage patties for 1 day or freeze them for up to 1 month. To cook the frozen patties, proceed with Step 2, cooking the patties for 7 to 9 minutes per side.

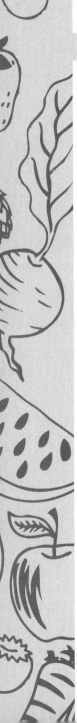

Beef and Spinach Breakfast Casserole

Prep time: 15 min • **Cook time:** 35–45 min • **Yield:** 6 servings

Ingredients	Directions
One 10-ounce package frozen spinach	**1** Preheat the oven to 375 degrees. Thaw the spinach in the microwave in 30-second intervals so you don't wind up cooking it. Drain in a colander with a weighted plate on top to press out the liquid.
1 pound ground beef	
10 eggs	**2** Fry the ground beef over medium heat until it's no longer pink. Drain.
2 cups whole milk	
Salt and pepper	**3** In a large bowl, mix the eggs and milk and beat well.
2 cups shredded cheese	
	4 Spread the beef on the bottom of a 13-x-9-inch glass or ceramic dish. Sprinkle with salt and pepper and cover with the spinach. Sprinkle that layer with salt and pepper. Pour in the egg mixture and sprinkle with salt and pepper. Top with the cheese.
	5 Bake for 35–45 minutes.

Per serving: Calories 589 (From Fat 414); Fat 46g (Saturated 21g); Cholesterol 417mg; Sodium 895mg; Carbohydrate 7g (Dietary Fiber 1g); Protein 34g.

Note: This dish keeps in the fridge for about 3 days. You can also cut it into single servings to store.

Vary It! Add extra flavor with chopped red or yellow bell peppers, chopped onions, or minced garlic. You can also substitute sausage for the ground beef.

The advantages of pastured eggs

Research shows that pastured eggs are the healthiest eggs available. They're better than even organic cage-free eggs. Studies have shown that chickens that spend most or all of their lives outdoors produce eggs that have

✔ ⅔ more vitamin A

✔ 2 times more omega-3 fatty acids

✔ 3 times more vitamin E

✔ 5 times more vitamin D

✔ 7 times more beta carotene

All of this over regular supermarket eggs. The best place to buy pastured eggs is from a local farmer.

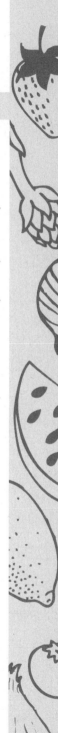

Chorizo and Pepper Jack Muffin-Tin Frittatas

Prep time: 35 min • **Cook time:** 15 min • **Yield:** 12 frittatas

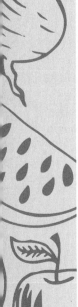

Ingredients	Directions
8 large eggs	*1* Adjust the oven rack to the lower-middle position and preheat the oven to 425 degrees.
¼ cup half and half	
½ teaspoon pepper	*2* Whisk the eggs, half and half, pepper, and ¼ teaspoon of the salt in a large bowl.
¾ teaspoon salt, divided	
1 tablespoon olive oil	*3* Heat the oil in 12-inch nonstick skillet over medium heat until it's shimmering. Add the chorizo, potatoes, onion, and remaining salt. Cook, stirring occasionally, until the potatoes are tender, about 10 to 15 minutes.
8 ounces Spanish style chorizo sausage, quartered lengthwise and sliced thin	
8 ounces Yukon gold potatoes, quartered lengthwise and sliced thin	*4* Stir in the garlic and cook until fragrant, about 30 seconds. Transfer the mixture to a bowl and let cool for 15 minutes. Stir in the cheese.
1 large onion, finely chopped	*5* Generously spray a 12-cup nonstick muffin tin with olive oil spray. Divide the chorizo mixture evenly among the muffin cups. Using a ladle, evenly distribute the egg mixture over the filling.
2 cloves garlic, minced	
6 ounces pepper jack cheese, shredded (1½ cups)	
	6 Bake until the frittatas are lightly puffed and just set in the center, about 9 to 11 minutes. Transfer the muffin tin to a wire rack and let cool for 10 minutes.
	7 Run a plastic knife around the edges of the frittatas if necessary to loosen them from the muffin tin. Gently remove the frittatas and serve.

Per serving: *Calories 178 (From Fat 108); Fat 12g (Saturated 5g); Cholesterol 158mg; Sodium 420mg; Carbohydrate 7g (Dietary Fiber 1g); Protein 12g.*

Note: You can prepare the egg and chorizo mixtures up to a day in advance and refrigerate them. You can also freeze them for up to a month or refrigerate some of the frittatas for 3 to 4 days for a grab-and-go option.

Vary It! Instead of chorizo and pepper jack, try using one of these filling combinations: asparagus and goat cheese, mushrooms and Gruyère, or red bell peppers and cheddar.

5-Minute Spinach and Cheese Omelet

Prep time: 5 min • **Cook time:** 5 min • **Yield:** 1 omelet

Ingredients	Directions
1 small tomato	*1* Dice the tomato. Peel and pit the avocado and scoop out the flesh with a spoon. Place the avocado on a plate.
1 small avocado	
3 eggs	
½ tablespoon butter	*2* Preheat an omelet pan or skillet on medium heat. In a small bowl, crack the eggs and whip together.
2 ounces shredded cheddar cheese	
1 cup raw spinach leaves	*3* Melt the butter in the pan. Add the eggs. Use a spatula to gently push one cooked edge of the egg into the center of the pan while tilting the pan the opposite direction to allow the liquid egg to flow underneath. Continue this process with the other edges until no liquid remains and the egg is almost cooked through.
Salt to taste	
	4 When the egg is nearly cooked through, add the cheese and spinach to half the omelet. Fold the other half over the filling; remove the pan from the heat and let it sit about 30 seconds.
	5 Put the omelet on the plate next to the avocado and top with the tomatoes. Salt to taste.

Per serving: Calories 742 (From Fat 540); Fat 60g (Saturated 23g); Cholesterol 633mg; Sodium 673mg; Carbohydrate 18g (Dietary Fiber 11g); Protein 38g.

Tip: Shred the cheese yourself instead of buying it already shredded. Manufacturers add unwanted starches to keep the cheese from clumping. And chunk cheese is usually less expensive anyway!

Vary It! You can easily add onions, garlic, or pepper to your omelet as desired (though you may need a little longer than five minutes when cooking).

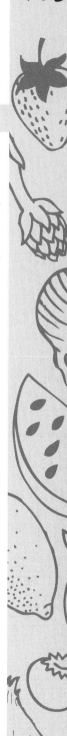

Piña Colada Smoothie

Prep time: 20 min • **Yield:** Three 2-cup servings

Ingredients	Directions
1 cup unsweetened coconut milk	*1* Blend the coconut milk and the protein powder in a blender until the powder dissolves.
⅓ cup whey protein powder	
2 cups frozen pineapple chunks	*2* Add the remaining ingredients and blend until smooth.
2 small bananas, roughly chopped (about 1½ cups)	
1½ cups plain whole-milk yogurt	
¼ cup raw macadamia nuts	

Per serving: Calories 731 (From Fat 423); Fat 47g (Saturated 18g); Cholesterol 90mg; Sodium 247mg; Carbohydrate 44g (Dietary Fiber 3g); Protein 33g.

Almond & Banana Smoothie

Prep time: 2 min • **Yield:** Two 2½-cup servings

Ingredients	Directions
½ cup apple juice	*1* Blend the apple juice, yogurt, and protein powder in a blender until the powder dissolves.
1½ cups plain yogurt	
⅓ cup whey protein powder	*2* Add the almond butter and blend until smooth.
¼ cup almond butter	
3 small bananas, frozen for at least 2 hours, roughly chopped (about 2¼ cups)	*3* Add the banana and blend until smooth.

Per serving: Calories 596 (From Fat 189); Fat 21g (Saturated 6g); Cholesterol 113mg; Sodium 267mg; Carbohydrate 61g (Dietary Fiber 7g); Protein 46g.

The Hangover Smoothie

Prep time: 3 min • **Yield:** 2 servings

Ingredients	Directions
1 cup apple juice	**1** Blend the apple juice, protein powder, and almonds until the powder dissolves.
⅓ cup hemp protein powder	
¼ cup raw almonds	**2** Add the remaining ingredients and blend until smooth.
1 small banana, frozen for at least 2 hours, roughly chopped (¾ cups)	
2 tablespoons ground flaxseeds	
½ cup frozen blueberries	

Per serving: Calories 388 (From Fat 171); Fat 19g (Saturated 1g); Cholesterol 0mg; Sodium 18mg; Carbohydrate 46g (Dietary Fiber 12g); Protein 17g.

Gingersnap Smoothie

Prep time: 4 min • **Yield:** One 2-cup serving

Ingredients	Directions
2 small bananas, frozen for at least 2 hours, roughly chopped (about 1½ cups)	**1** Blend all the ingredients in a blender until smooth.
½ cup frozen peaches	
1 cup almond milk	
½ cup chai tea	
2 tablespoons chopped fresh ginger	
⅓ cup whey protein powder	

Per serving: Calories 714 (From Fat 90); Fat 10g (Saturated 3g); Cholesterol 210mg; Sodium 335mg; Carbohydrate 89g (Dietary Fiber 8g); Protein 74g.

Hidden Veggie Smoothie

Prep time: 5 min • **Yield:** Two 2-cup servings

Ingredients	Directions
1½ cups almond milk	**1** Blend the milk, both powders, and almonds in a blender until the powders dissolve.
¼ cup whey protein powder	
¼ cup hemp protein powder	**2** Add the remaining ingredients and blend until smooth.
1 ounce raw almonds (about 25 nuts)	
1 medium banana, frozen for at least 2 hours, roughly chopped (about 1 cup)	
½ cup frozen blueberries	
½ cup frozen kale	
½ avocado	

Per serving: Calories 402 (From Fat 289); Fat 17g (Saturated 2g); Cholesterol 66mg; Sodium 107mg; Carbohydrate 33g (Dietary Fiber 11g); Protein 35g.

Chapter 9

Easy Everyday Entrees

In This Chapter

▶ Focusing on quality ingredients

▶ Generating hearty salad ideas that will serve as a meal

▶ Creating wheat-free meals everyone will love

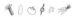
*E*liminating wheat from your diet doesn't mean that you're on a diet; yes, it's a lifestyle change, but you don't have to give up all your favorite foods. You just have to rethink some of them. Actually, you'll find that most wheat ingredients have a wheat-free replacement, allowing you to enjoy many of the entrees that you're accustomed to eating.

In this chapter, we provide several delicious entree recipes that the entire family will enjoy. By substituting a few wheat-free ingredients here and there, you discover a whole new way of cooking. These wheat-free entrees not only please the palate but also provide everyone in your house with healthy food.

Fixing Healthy and Tasty Main Dishes

The recipes in this chapter are a blueprint of what all your entree recipes will look like in the future. The more you prepare them, the better your understanding of what to use and how to use it as you produce a wheat-free masterpiece. The key lies in working with nutrient-rich, quality ingredients. If you read through the ingredient lists in this chapter, you'll find a familiar friend: olive oil. Olive oil has been shown to lower blood pressure, lower LDL (bad cholesterol), and prevent certain cancers. A friend you may be less familiar with is avocado oil (you can find it in the Spaghetti Squash with Meat Sauce recipe). Similar in health benefits to olive oil, avocado oil improves heart health, aids in weight loss, and helps prevent cancer.

One important thing to consider with oils are their *smoke points,* or the maximum temperatures you can heat them to before they smoke and begin to break down and lose nutritional value (and flavor). Generally speaking, the smoke point of olive oil is 410 degrees Fahrenheit; for extra-virgin olive oil, it's around 400 degrees, and refined avocado oil is 520 degrees. Our recipes keep the oil below these temperatures, so enjoy without guilt.

Another important factor is meat quality. Grain-fed animals and farmed animals are often sick and don't provide the omega-3 fatty acids that grass-fed cows and wild-caught fish do. When you use grass-fed beef, wild salmon, and air-chilled organic chicken whenever possible, you're guaranteed the best benefits those meats have to offer. They're a little bit more expensive, but they're definitely worth it. (Never heard of air-chilled chicken? Head to the nearby sidebar "Checkin' out chicken labels.")

Checkin' out chicken labels

Understanding all the different chicken classifications you see at the store can be very confusing. Even the regulations that define these categories leave a lot of wiggle room for the manufacturers. The only true way to know how the chicken was raised is to buy from a local farmer whose farm you've visited. Truly organic, humane farmers love to share their craft, and the visit can be quite enlightening. But if that's not an option, here's a breakdown of the basic labels you may find on chicken in the grocery store, starting with the best:

✔ **Organic:** This is really the only label that has any laws behind it. The chickens are fed 100 percent organic feed. They have to be *free-range,* which means they are probably allowed to roam in a pasture, and given no antibiotics. Because regulators scrutinize the organic label, most organic farmers confirm to the strictest of rules.

✔ **Kosher or halal:** These terms refer to Jewish or Muslim law, respectively. Birds with this label tend to be treated more humanely, and the farmers are held to higher standards than non-kosher or non-halal farmers. For example, they must check for sick animals and kill by hand rather than by machine.

✔ **Pastured:** This terminology isn't strictly legally regulated, so you need to do a bit of research into the manufacturer to find out what it means for that given brand. It implies that the birds can roam free and feed on their natural diet. They may additionally be fed grains (which aren't part of their traditional diet), but on the whole they're much happier and healthier chickens than conventionally raised birds.

✔ **Air-chilled:** The chickens are cooled with air rather than in water.

✔ **Natural:** The term *natural* refers only to what manufacturers have added after the birds are slaughtered, such as flavorings, colorings, or brines. It gives you no information about how the chicken was raised.

One final note: By law, no chickens can be given hormones, so if you see a product touting "no hormones," know that that's not anything special.

Don't be scared off by the higher price tag on quality proteins. You save lots of money by not buying wheat and all the products associated with it, so you can redirect some of this money to increase the meat and fish budget.

As you whip up the entrees in this chapter, consider doubling the recipes. Cooking a larger batch allows you to have enough leftovers for lunch the next day; you can't beat the price, the time it takes to prepare it, or the quality of food. Many foods with a lot of different seasonings taste better the next day because the flavors have blended together. Doubling the ingredients in the recipes also allows you to freeze extra servings for snacks and meals for a later date.

Making a Meal of Salads

The best way to make a hearty entree salad is to incorporate a protein. Adding beef, chicken, or seafood to any salad makes you feel like you've had a full dinner every time. Make a little extra and set some aside without the dressing so you can enjoy a salad lunch the next day.

If you're planning on taking extra salad to school or work the next day, place the salad dressing in a separate container so your salad remains crisp.

One of the best things about salads is that they're an easy meal to put together. Always keep some of these salad staples on hand: avocadoes, tomatoes, spinach, green leaf or romaine lettuce, bell peppers, broccoli, strawberries, mandarin oranges, nuts, cheese, and the meat of your choice. Salads are easy to keep wheat-free; just don't add croutons.

Leaf through the following suggestions to create a healthy, great-tasting meal salad:

- **Use organic produce and high-quality meat whenever possible.** Doing so ensures that your salad is free of insecticides, pesticides, hormones, and antibiotics. (We explain the best meat options in the preceding section.)

- **Thoroughly rinse the produce with water.** Using soap can leave your ingredients tasting soapy. Pat all of your leafy greens dry; the more water left on your salad fixings, the less crisp your salad will be.

- **Toss the salad carefully, allowing the dressing to cover all ingredients.**

Chicken-Stuffed Poblano Peppers

Prep time: 30 min • **Cook time:** 40–45 min • **Yield:** 4 servings

Ingredients	Directions
4 poblano peppers	*1* Preheat the broiler to high with the oven rack about 4 inches from the heating element. Line a large rimmed baking sheet with foil.
½ a medium white onion, chopped	
½ cup sour cream	*2* Place the poblanos on the baking sheet and broil them, turning every few minutes, until blackened all over (5 to 8 minutes). Let cool.
1 large clove garlic, chopped	
1 teaspoon dried oregano, crumbled	*3* Peel off the poblano skins (you may want to wear rubber gloves). Make a slit in the long side of the pepper and carefully remove the seeds and membranes, leaving the stems on. Return the poblanos to the baking sheet.
½ teaspoon salt, plus more to taste	
2 cups shredded rotisserie chicken, preferably dark meat	*4* Reduce the oven heat to 375 degrees. Puree the onion, sour cream, garlic, oregano, and ½ teaspoon of salt in a food processor.
2 cups grated Monterrey Jack cheese, divided	*5* Cook the mixture in a 12-inch skillet over medium heat, stirring frequently, until the liquid has evaporated, 8 to 11 minutes. Remove the pan from the heat and set aside.
1 teaspoon ground cumin	
Generous pinch ground cinnamon	*6* In a bowl, mix the chicken, 1 cup of the cheese, the cumin, cinnamon, apricots, and pumpkin seeds. Season with salt to taste.
¼ cup dried apricots, chopped	*7* Divide the filling among the peppers, being careful not to tear them (some filling will still be exposed). Top with the sour cream sauce.
¼ cup pumpkin seeds, unsalted	
	8 Bake the stuffed peppers for 20 to 30 minutes until the cheese is melted and bubbly. Top with the remaining cheese and broil until the cheese is completely melted, about 2 minutes. Serve.

Per serving: Calories 646 (From Fat 432); Fat 48g (Saturated 208g); Cholesterol 20mg; Sodium 1,281mg; Carbohydrate 13g (Dietary Fiber 2g); Protein 44g.

Vary It! Add one 28-ounce can of red tomatoes in Step 4 and substitute cheddar and cilantro for the cinnamon, apricots, and pumpkin seeds. Two cheeses are better than one!

Spicy Lime Chicken with Black Bean and Avocado Salad

Prep time: 15 min, plus marinating time • **Cook time:** 8–13 min • **Yield:** 4 servings

Ingredients	Directions
⅓ cup lime juice	**1** Preheat the grill to medium high heat.
½ cup chopped fresh cilantro leaves	**2** Whisk the lime juice, cilantro, oil, chiles, adobo sauce, honey, garlic, cumin, ½ teaspoon of salt, and ¼ teaspoon of pepper in a small bowl. Transfer ¼ cup of this mixture to a large bowl.
¼ cup olive oil	
2 chipotle peppers in adobo, roughly chopped	
2 tablespoons adobo sauce	**3** Toss the chicken with the lime juice mixture in the large bowl. Season with the remaining salt and pepper. Marinate chicken in the refrigerator for 15 minutes while the grill is preheating.
1 tablespoon honey	
3 medium cloves garlic, minced	
2 teaspoons ground cumin	
1 teaspoon salt, plus more to taste	**4** Toss the beans, scallions, bell pepper, and avocado with another ¼ cup of the lime juice mixture in another bowl. Season with salt and pepper to taste.
½ teaspoon pepper, plus more to taste	
8 boneless, skinless chicken thighs or 4 boneless, skinless chicken breasts	**5** Grill the chicken over a hot fire on both sides until cooked through, 5 to 6 minutes per side. Transfer the chicken to a serving platter and drizzle with the remaining lime juice mixture (about ½ cup).
Two 16-ounce cans black beans, drained and rinsed	
½ cup chopped scallions	
1 red bell pepper, thinly sliced	**6** Slice the chicken and serve immediately topped with the black bean and avocado salad.
1 ripe avocado, pitted, peeled, and thinly sliced	
Lime wedges for serving	

Per serving: Calories 612 (From Fat 216); Fat 24g (Saturated 4g); Cholesterol 72g; Sodium 1,256mg; Carbohydrate 67g (Dietary Fiber 14g); Protein 44g.

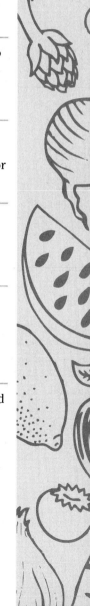

Easy Baked Salmon with Tomatoes and Herbs

Prep time: 15 min • **Cook time:** 25 min • **Yield:** 4 servings

Ingredients	Directions
Four 6-to-8-ounce skinless salmon fillets	**1** Preheat the oven to 400 degrees.
1 teaspoon salt, divided	**2** Sprinkle the salmon with ½ teaspoon of salt. In a medium bowl, blend the tomatoes, shallots, lemon juice, oregano, thyme, remaining salt, and 2 tablespoons of olive oil.
One 14-ounce can chopped tomatoes, drained	
1 shallot, chopped	
2 tablespoons lemon juice	**3** Place ½ teaspoon each of the butter and remaining olive oil on a piece of aluminum foil and top with a salmon fillet on top. Spoon ¼ of the tomato mixture over the salmon.
1 teaspoon dried oregano	
1 teaspoon dried thyme	
2 teaspoons butter	**4** Fold the sides of the foil over the contents, covering completely, and seal the packet tightly. Repeat Steps 3 and 4 with the remaining butter, olive oil, salmon, and tomato mixture and place the packets on a large, heavy baking sheet.
3 tablespoons plus 1 teaspoon olive oil, divided	
	5 Bake until the salmon is just cooked through, 20 to 25 minutes. Open the packets and slide the salmon with sauce onto plates.

Per serving: Calories 404 (From Fat 189); Fat 21g (Saturated 4.5g); Cholesterol 83mg; Sodium 1,788mg; Carbohydrate 9g (Dietary Fiber 1g); Protein 45g.

Spaghetti Squash with Meat Sauce

Prep time: 35 min • **Cook time:** 40–50 min • **Yield:** 4 servings

Ingredients	Directions
1 spaghetti squash (about 1½ pounds) 1 small onion, finely chopped 2 teaspoons butter or avocado oil 2 cloves garlic, peeled and minced One 28-ounce can whole peeled tomatoes ½ tablespoon salt 1 teaspoon dried oregano ½ teaspoon red pepper flakes 5 sprigs fresh thyme 1½ pounds ground beef Fresh basil leaves	*1* Preheat the oven to 400 degrees. Halve the squash lengthwise; scoop out and discard the seeds. Place the squash, flesh side down, in a 9-by-13-inch glass baking dish. Pour water into the dish until it's halfway up the squash. Bake 40 to 50 minutes until the squash begins to brown.
	2 While the squash bakes, sauté the onions in the butter or oil in a large pot over medium heat for 5 minutes. Add the butter, garlic, tomatoes, salt, oregano, pepper flakes, and thyme and cover; reduce the heat to low and cook for 30 minutes.
	3 Cook the ground beef in a frying pan over medium heat until it's no longer pink. Set aside.
	4 Remove the thyme stems from the sauce. Puree with a stick blender until smooth and then add the beef.
	5 Remove the squash from oven. When it's cool enough to handle, scrape the flesh crosswise with a fork to pull squash strands from shell and place in a serving bowl. Top them with the sauce and garnish with fresh basil.

Per serving: Calories 574 (From Fat 288); Fat 32g (Saturated 13g); Cholesterol 156mg; Sodium 1,744mg; Carbohydrate 22g (Dietary Fiber 5g); Protein 49g.

Tip: Double the sauce; it goes fast!

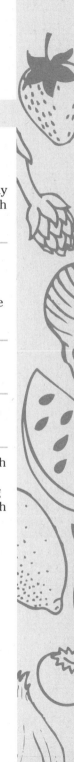

Chicken Pot Pie

Prep time: 10 min • **Cook time:** 25–30 min • **Yield:** 8 servings

Ingredients	*Directions*
Biscuit Topping (see the following recipe)	*1* Prepare the Biscuit Topping. While the biscuits are baking, bring the stock, bay leaves, and thyme to a boil in a large pot or Dutch oven over medium-high heat. Add the potatoes, celery, peppers, and garlic. Cover and cook for 5 minutes.
5 cups chicken stock	
2 bay leaves	
2 sprigs fresh thyme	
1½ cups diced unpeeled round red potatoes	*2* Add the carrots. Cover and cook for 3 minutes. Add the mushrooms; cover and cook for 5 minutes.
½ cup chopped celery	
½ cup chopped red bell pepper	
1 clove garlic, minced	*3* In a medium bowl, whisk the flour, salt, pepper, and heavy cream and add to the pot. Add the peas and cook over medium heat for 3 minutes or until the gravy is thickened and bubbly, stirring constantly.
¾ cup thinly sliced carrots	
1 cup sliced fresh mushrooms	
6 tablespoons coconut flour	
1 teaspoon salt	*4* Remove the pot from the heat and add the chicken. Top with two of the biscuits and serve.
1 teaspoon pepper	
1 cup heavy whipping cream	
½ cup frozen green peas	
1 store-bought rotisserie chicken, meat removed from bone and skin discarded	

Biscuit Topping

Ingredients	Directions
2 cups almond flour 2 teaspoons baking powder ½ teaspoon salt ⅛ teaspoon garlic powder 1 cup whole milk 1½ tablespoons melted butter	*1* Preheat the oven to 400 degrees. In a medium bowl, combine the flour, baking powder, salt, and garlic powder. *2* Stir in the milk and butter just until the flour mixture is moistened. *3* Spoon the biscuits evenly onto a large baking sheet lined with parchment paper until you have about 16 biscuits. Bake for 20 minutes.

Per serving: Calories 545 (From Fat 315); Fat 35g (Saturated 10g); Cholesterol 103mg; Sodium 1,072mg; Carbohydrate 27g (Dietary Fiber 7g); Protein 34g.

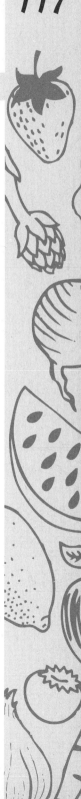

Lemon Drumsticks

Prep time: 30 min, plus brining time • **Cook time:** 20 min • **Yield:** About 6 servings

Ingredients	Directions
⅓ cup kosher salt	*1* Put 6 cups of water and the kosher salt in a large bowl; dissolve. Add the chicken, covering it in the brine, and refrigerate for about 1½ hours.
1½ to 2 pounds chicken drumsticks	
Salt and pepper for seasoning	*2* Preheat the broiler with the top rack about 5 inches from the heating element.
¼ cup extra-virgin olive oil	
4 cloves garlic, minced	*3* Remove the chicken from the brine and discard the brining liquid. Dry the chicken thoroughly with paper towels and season with salt and pepper.
1 cup lemon juice	
1½ teaspoons dried thyme	
	4 Heat the olive oil and garlic in a medium skillet over low heat until it starts to sizzle but not color, about 30 seconds. Remove from the heat and add the lemon juice and thyme. Set aside.
	5 Broil the chicken on a broiler pan for 14 minutes or until it's dark golden brown and registers 170 to 175 degrees on an instant-read thermometer. Keep an eye on the broiling chicken and turn it as necessary.
	6 Set aside half the lemon sauce. Roll the chicken in the remaining lemon sauce in the skillet to coat completely. Serve the chicken warm drizzled with the reserved sauce.

Per serving: Calories 303 (From Fat 180); Fat 20g (Saturated 4g); Cholesterol 147mg; Sodium 4,854mg; Carbohydrate 4g (Dietary Fiber 0g); Protein 26g.

Tip: This recipe is also tasty eaten cold right out of the refrigerator.

Almond-Flax-Crusted Chicken Tenders

Prep time: 15 min • **Cook time:** 20–30 min • **Yield:** 4 servings

Ingredients	*Directions*
1½ pounds chicken tenders	**1** Preheat the oven to 350 degrees.
½ cup almond meal	
3 tablespoons ground flax	**2** Rinse and pat the chicken dry. Combine the almond meal and flax in a zip-top bag and mix evenly.
2 tablespoons extra-virgin olive oil	
2 tablespoons almond butter	**3** In bowl, combine the olive oil, almond butter, lemon juice, and all spices and herbs. Add the chicken and toss to coat.
2 teaspoons lemon juice	
2 teaspoons sea salt	
⅛ teaspoon cayenne pepper	**4** Place the chicken two to three tenders at a time in the zip-top bag and shake to coat with the almond meal. Place the coated tenders on a baking tray.
2 teaspoons fresh parsley	
½ teaspoon paprika	
2 teaspoons fresh thyme	**5** Bake for about 20 to 30 minutes or until an instant-read thermometer reads 168 degrees.
1 tablespoon finely chopped fresh onion	

Per serving: Calories 620 (From Fat 378); Fat 42g (Saturated 7g); Cholesterol 70mg; Sodium 1,695mg; Carbohydrate 32g (Dietary Fiber 4g); Protein 31g.

Tip: You can leave the chicken in the marinade for up to 24 hours to prepare the dish in advance or enhance the flavor. You can also freeze the chicken in the marinade for use at a later date; just thaw it and apply the almond mixture as instructed in Step 4.

Note: You can buy almond meal in the grocery store or make it at home from almonds in a food processor or high-powered blender.

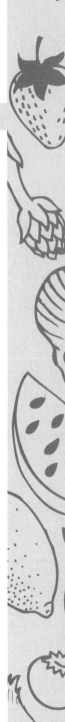

Beef in a Leaf

Prep time: 7 min • **Cook time:** 10 min • **Yield:** 4 servings

Ingredients	Directions
5 cups rice noodles	**1** Prepare the rice noodles according to the package directions. Drain and set aside.
2 tablespoons olive oil	
1 pound sirloin or flank steak, cut into 2-inch-x-¼-inch strips	**2** Heat the oil in a large skillet. Add the beef and cook until browned, about 5 to 6 minutes.
¼ cup raw coconut aminos	**3** Add the coconut aminos, vinegar, honey, and pepper flakes. Cook, stirring constantly, for about 1 minute. Add the cooked noodles and toss to coat. Cook until the noodles are heated through, about 1 minute longer.
¼ cup balsamic vinegar	
⅛ cup honey	
½ teaspoon crushed red pepper flakes	
1 head red leaf lettuce separated, washed, and patted dry	**4** Arrange the lettuce leaves on a platter. Spoon the beef mixture onto each lettuce leaf. Roll up and eat.

Per serving: Calories 564 (From Fat 144); Fat 16g (Saturated 5g); Cholesterol 53mg; Sodium 476mg; Carbohydrate 72g (Dietary Fiber 3g); Protein 28g.

Tip: You can add sweet red chili sauce or sriracha hot chili sauce as desired to the finished product.

Note: Coconut aminos come from the sap of a coconut tree. You can find them in health food stores, in vitamin shops, and online.

Greek Salad with Shrimp

Prep time: 15 min • **Cook time:** 10 min • **Yield:** About 4 servings

Ingredients	Directions
Juice of 1 lemon, plus 2 teaspoons	*1* Bring the juice of 1 lemon, the bay leaves, 1 teaspoon of the salt, the peppercorns, Old Bay, and 4 cups of water to a boil in a large pot for 2 minutes. Remove from the heat.
2 bay leaves	
2 teaspoons salt	
1 teaspoon black peppercorns	
1 teaspoon Old Bay seasoning	*2* Add the shrimp to the pot; cover and steep until the shrimp are firm and pink, about 7 minutes. Drain the shrimp and plunge them into ice water. Drain the shrimp and peel the shells.
1 pound unpeeled raw extra large shrimp	
1 cucumber, peeled and sliced ¼-inch thick	
1 large green bell pepper, diced	*3* Place the cucumber, peppers, tomatoes, onion, feta, capers, and remaining lemon juice in a large bowl.
1 pint grape tomatoes, halved	
1 bunch (about 4) green onions, white parts only, sliced	*4* In a lidded container, vigorously shake the garlic, oregano, mustard, vinegar, remaining salt, pepper, and oil for 30 seconds. Pour the vinaigrette over the vegetables, add the shrimp, and toss lightly. Serve at room temperature.
½ pound feta cheese, ½-inch diced	
2 tablespoons capers, drained	
2 cloves garlic, minced	
1 teaspoon dried oregano	
½ teaspoon Dijon mustard	
¼ cup red wine vinegar or sherry vinegar	
½ cup extra-virgin olive oil	

Per serving: Calories 405 (From Fat 243); Fat 27g (Saturated 9g); Cholesterol 185mg; Sodium 2,801mg; Carbohydrate 16g (Dietary Fiber 4g); Protein 29g.

Vary It! Substitute avocado and tomato for the feta cheese and cucumber in the dressing.

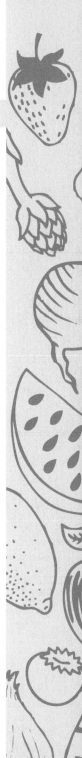

Southwestern Caesar Salad

Prep time: 10 min • **Cook time:** 14–18 min • **Yield:** 8 servings

Ingredients	Directions
2 pounds chicken breasts	**1** Preheat the oven to 350 degrees with the rack about 5 inches from the heating element.
1 teaspoon pepper, plus more for seasoning	
1 teaspoon salt, plus more for seasoning	**2** Place the chicken breasts on a broiler pan and season with a bit of salt and pepper. Cook for 14 to 18 minutes. Set aside.
1 large clove garlic, peeled	
4 oil-packed anchovy fillets, drained	**3** In a blender or food processor, puree the garlic, anchovies, chipotles, and mustard. Add the cheese, egg, lime juice, and 1 teaspoon each of pepper and salt. Process until smooth.
1 canned chipotle pepper, stems and seeds removed	
1 tablespoon Dijon mustard	
1 cup grated Parmigiano-Reggiano cheese	**4** With the blender or processor running, slowly add the olive oil in a thin stream. If the dressing becomes too thick, add a tablespoon of water and continue until all the oil is incorporated.
1 pasteurized egg	
Juice from 3 limes	**5** Taste and adjust seasoning with salt and pepper to taste.
1½ cups extra-virgin olive oil	
2 to 3 heads romaine lettuce	**6** Toss the lettuce with the dressing. Cut the chicken into thin strips and add to the salad. Garnish with the bell peppers, pine nuts, or poblanos (if desired).
Roasted red bell peppers (optional)	
Toasted pine nuts (optional)	
Roasted poblano peppers (optional)	

Per serving: *Calories 612 (From Fat 441); Fat 49g (Saturated 9g); Cholesterol 129mg; Sodium 576mg; Carbohydrate 2g (Dietary Fiber 1g); Protein 41g.*

Tip: For even more chipotle flavor, you can add a drop or two of the adobo sauce the chipotles come canned in to the sauce mixture in Step 3.

Note: Pasteurized eggs can be used for any recipe that calls for raw eggs, like eggnog, meringue, hollandaise sauce, or Caesar dressings. They've gone through a process to ensure any bacteria or viruses are destroyed. All liquid eggs are pasteurized; in-shell eggs that have been pasteurized will be stamped with a red P.

Chapter 10

One-Pot Meals

*W*hat better way to enjoy a meal than with very little clean-up after you eat? Sometimes knowing you don't have a slew of pans to scrub after you devour a meal can make the food taste that much better! What's more, wheat doesn't usually play a big role in one-pot meals, so many of these recipes may look very similar to what you already enjoy.

Singing the Praises of One-Pot Meals

Traditionally, Americans think of one-pot recipes as slow cooker dishes. Although slow cooker recipes do make for easy clean-up and tasty meals, they typically require hours of cooking. In this chapter, we've assembled a sampling of one-pot meals that don't take nearly as long. As advertised, they require only a large pot or Dutch oven.

One-pot meals are great for those who have trouble getting everything cooked and hot on the table at the same time. And combining all the different ingredients in one pot allows the flavors to meld in a way that serving them separately on a plate can't accomplish.

One-pot meals also give you the flexibility to substitute ingredients to accommodate different tastes in your household. Feel free to double the vegetables or spices as desired or just double the whole recipe and enjoy leftovers the next day.

To make things even easier at dinnertime, try precutting the ingredients in the morning so you just have to dump them into the pot that night. This way, you have more time to catch up with the family after a long day at work or school.

Chili Surprise

Prep time: 15 min • **Cook time:** 1 hr • **Yield:** 4 to 6 servings

Ingredients	Directions
½ pound ground bison	*1* Heat a large pot over high heat. Brown the bison, stirring often, for 5 minutes.
1 large onion, finely chopped	
1 large carrot, finely chopped	*2* Add the onion and carrot and cook until they begin to soften, about 5 minutes. Add ½ cup of water to deglaze the pan. Scrape the brown bits from the bottom of the pan until the water evaporates.
½ head cauliflower, finely chopped	
1 medium green bell pepper, finely chopped	
3 large cloves garlic, finely chopped	*3* Add the cauliflower, bell pepper, and garlic to the pan and cook until the vegetables begin to soften, about 5 minutes.
2 teaspoons ground cumin	
2 tablespoons chili powder	*4* Add the cumin, chili powder, vinegar, tomatoes, beans, and chipotle pepper and 1 cup of water. Bring to a boil. Reduce to a simmer and cover.
1 tablespoon apple cider vinegar	
One 15-ounce can no-salt-added diced tomatoes	*5* Cook, stirring occasionally, until the vegetables are fork tender, about 45 minutes. Serve garnished with the cilantro.
One 28-ounce can no-salt-added crushed tomatoes	
One 15-ounce can no-salt-added kidney beans, drained and rinsed	
1 chipotle pepper in adobo sauce, finely chopped	
½ cup loosely packed fresh cilantro leaves, chopped	

Per serving: Calories 218 (From Fat 36); Fat 4g (Saturated 1g); Cholesterol 21mg; Sodium 552mg; Carbohydrate 34g (Dietary Fiber 11g); Protein 17g.

Shrimp with Tarragon Broth

Prep time: 5 min • **Cook time:** 25–27 min • **Yield:** 4 servings

Ingredients	Directions
2 tablespoons olive oil	**1** In a large pot, heat the olive oil over medium-low heat. Add the onion, celery, garlic, and salt. Cook, stirring occasionally, until the vegetables start to soften, about 10 minutes.
1 onion, peeled and chopped	
2 ribs celery, chopped	
2 cloves garlic, peeled and minced	**2** Add the tarragon, clam juice, tomatoes, and chicken stock. Bring to a boil. Reduce the heat and simmer for 10 minutes.
¾ teaspoon salt	
1¼ teaspoon dried tarragon	
1 cup bottled clam juice	**3** Stir the shrimp into the soup. Cook, stirring occasionally, until the shrimp is just done, 3 to 5 minutes. Stir in the pepper and serve.
One 15-ounce can diced tomatoes with their juice	
One 32-ounce box of chicken stock	
1½ pounds medium shrimp, shelled and deveined	
¼ teaspoon pepper	

Per serving: Calories 331 (From Fat 99); Fat 11g (Saturated 2g); Cholesterol 221mg; Sodium 2,046mg; Carbohydrate 26g (Dietary Fiber 2g); Protein 31g.

Tip: If you've never deveined shrimp before, check out Figure 10-1.

Cleaning and Deveining Shrimp

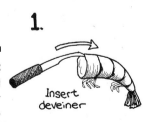

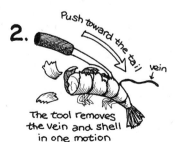

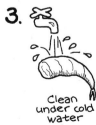

Figure 10-1: Cleaning and deveining shrimp.

1. Insert deveiner

2. Push toward the tail — vein — The tool removes the vein and shell in one motion

3. Clean under cold water

Illustration by Elizabeth Kurtzman

Tuscan Bean Stew

Prep time: 10 min • **Cook time:** about 1 hr • **Yield:** 8 to 10 servings

Ingredients	Directions
1 tablespoon extra-virgin olive oil, plus more for garnish	**1** Heat the olive oil and pancetta in a large Dutch oven over medium heat. Cook, stirring occasionally, until the pancetta is lightly browned and its fat has rendered, about 6 to 10 minutes.
6 ounces pancetta, ¼-inch chopped	
1 large onion, medium chopped (about 1½ cups)	**2** Add the onion, celery, and carrots. Cook, stirring occasionally, until they're softened and lightly browned, about 10 to 16 minutes. Stir in the garlic and cook until fragrant, about 1 minute.
2 medium pieces celery, ½-inch chopped (about ¾ cup)	
2 medium carrots, peeled and ½-inch chopped (about 1 cup)	**3** Stir in the broth, 2 cups of water, the beans, bay leaves, tomatoes, and greens. Increase the heat to high and bring to a simmer.
8 medium cloves garlic, minced (about 3 tablespoons)	
3 cups chicken broth	**4** Reduce the heat and simmer until the vegetables and greens are fully tender, about 20 to 25 minutes.
Four 15-ounce cans of cannellini beans, drained and rinsed well	
2 medium bay leaves	**5** Remove the pot from the stove and submerge the rosemary. Cover and let stand 15 minutes. Discard the bay leaves and rosemary.
One 15-ounce can diced tomatoes, drained and rinsed	
1 pound kale or collard greens, thick stems trimmed and leaves 1-inch chopped	**6** Season with salt and pepper to taste. Serve lightly drizzled with olive oil.
One 3-inch sprig fresh rosemary	
Salt and pepper to taste	

Per serving: Calories 278 (From Fat 72); Fat 8g (Saturated 3g); Cholesterol 12mg; Sodium 874mg; Carbohydrate 35g (Dietary Fiber 10g); Protein 16g.

Traditional Yankee Pot Roast

Prep time: 20 min • **Cook time:** 3 hr • **Yield:** 8–10 servings

Ingredients	Directions
2 teaspoons avocado oil **4 pounds boneless chuck roast, trimmed** **1 tablespoon kosher salt** **1 tablespoon pepper**	*1* Preheat the oven to 300 degrees. Heat the avocado oil in a large Dutch oven over medium-high heat. Sprinkle the roast with the salt and pepper and brown it on all sides for about 8 minutes total. Remove the roast and set it aside.
2 cups coarsely chopped sweet onions	*2* Sauté the onions for 8 minutes or until browned. Put the roast back in the pan.
2 cups low-sodium beef broth **¼ cup low-sugar ketchup** **2 tablespoons gluten-free Worcestershire sauce**	*3* In a medium bowl, combine the broth, ketchup, and Worcestershire. Pour the mixture over the roast, add the tomatoes, and bring to a simmer.
1 cup chopped plum tomatoes **1 pound small red potatoes** **1 pound carrots, peeled and 1-inch chopped**	*4* Cover and roast in the oven for 2½ hours or until tender. Add the potatoes and carrots. Cover and roast an additional 30 minutes or until the vegetables are tender.

Per serving: Calories 658 (From Fat 360); Fat 40g (Saturated 16g); Cholesterol 181mg; Sodium 841mg; Carbohydrate 21g (Dietary Fiber 3g); Protein 51g.

Tip: If you cut against the grain, the meat will hold together and not shred. Figure 10-2 shows you how to do it.

Cutting Pot Roast Across the Grain

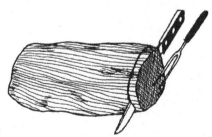

Figure 10-2: The best way to cut a pot roast.

Illustration by Elizabeth Kurtzman

Chicken Mexican Soup

Prep time: 20 min • **Cook time:** 30 min • **Yield:** 8 servings

Ingredients	*Directions*
2 pounds chicken breast	*1* Heat the oven to 350 degrees with the rack about 5 inches from the heating element. Sprinkle the chicken breasts with salt and pepper, and cook them on a broiler pan for 14 to 18 minutes. Set aside.
Sprinkle of salt and pepper, plus more to taste	
1 tablespoon olive oil	
½ cup thinly sliced onion	*2* Heat the olive oil in a 3-quart or larger soup pot over medium heat. Add the onions and carrots, and sauté until they begin to soften, about 10 minutes.
1 cup thinly sliced carrot	
1 handful cilantro stems, rinsed and tied together	*3* Add the cilantro stems and the stock. Bring to a boil, reduce the heat to medium/low, and simmer for 15 minutes. While the soup is simmering, pit, peel, and chop the avocados and dice the chicken breasts.
2 quarts organic chicken stock	
2 avocados	
2 cups pico de gallo	*4* Remove the cilantro stems and season the soup with salt and pepper to taste. Keep over warm heat.
2 cups grated Monterey Jack cheese	
8 lime wedges	*5* Divide the diced chicken among 8 soup bowls. Ladle the soup over the chicken and top each bowl with ¼ cup of the cheese, ¼ cup of the pico de gallo, and ⅛ of the avocado. Use a squeeze of one lime wedge per serving.

Per serving: Calories 477 (From Fat 207); Fat 23g (Saturated 8g); Cholesterol 128mg; Sodium 1,065mg; Carbohydrate 17g (Dietary Fiber 4g); Protein 49g.

Tip: You can find a Pico de Gallo recipe in Chapter 12. You can use the leftover cilantro leaves in that recipe.

Note: This recipe tastes even better when you use homemade chicken stock rather than the store-bought type.

Chapter 11

Savory Vegetable Sides

In This Chapter

▶ Loading up on nutrient-dense vegetables

▶ Discovering great wheat-free vegetable side dishes to complement your entrees

Do side dishes become an afterthought when you're preparing dinner? If so, you're not alone. Most people don't think in terms of balance and diversifying flavors with their side dishes. Consequently, their sides become nutritionally empty, boring, and unimaginative. In this chapter, we provide you with some tasty, nutritionally packed, wheat-free side dishes that are sure to excite you come dinnertime (or anytime).

All these recipes are terrific wheat-free substitutes for the traditional sides that you've given up to improve your health. With collard greens, asparagus, Brussels sprouts, spinach, and kale at the center of our recipes, you're sure to reap the benefits of this nutrient explosion.

Checking out the Nutritional Prowess of Vegetables

If variety is the spice of life, then the recipes in this chapter will make your life plenty spicy (figuratively speaking, of course). *Variety* in this context means foods with a wide range of vitamin and mineral content.

Nutritionally speaking, here's what's happening in our wheat-free side dishes:

- **Asparagus:** This green, white, or purple vegetable is rich in vitamins A, B6, C, E, and K and in minerals such as folic acid, copper, and iron. The chromium in asparagus helps insulin move blood sugar into muscle cells, where it can be used for energy. The antioxidants and glutathione in asparagus help prevent cancer by eliminating free radicals and carcinogens.

- **Broccoli:** Generally regarded as one of the healthiest vegetables in the world, broccoli's cancer-fighting abilities are second to none. It provides a healthy dose of vitamins A, C, and K; folate; potassium; and even omega-3 fatty acids.

- **Brussels sprouts:** These baby cabbages belong in the same family as broccoli, collard greens, and kale. This nutritional superstar is loaded with vitamins C and A and beta carotene, helping to prevent cancer and heart disease. Brussels sprouts' high level of omega-3 fatty acids and anti-inflammatory effects help keep diseases at bay.

- **Cauliflower:** Cauliflower's cancer-fighting *phytochemicals* (naturally occurring chemical compounds) are capable of halting cancer growth in certain organs. Cauliflower also contains many B vitamins that help with carbohydrate metabolism, which assists in weight loss, and minerals such as copper, potassium, iron, and calcium.

- **Collard greens:** Collard greens pack a powerful punch in disease prevention. Their high levels of vitamins C and A and beta carotene bolster the immune system and assist in preventing cancer and heart disease. The folate, vitamin B6, and magnesium in collards contribute to an improvement in heart health. Plus, they provide a source of calcium.

- **Kale:** One of the hottest food topics today is the health-promoting aspects of kale. With its large quantities of vitamins A, C, K, and B6 and its phytochemicals, it's a formidable foe in the assault against disease. Potassium, also found in kale, helps control heart rate and blood pressure.

- **Spinach:** As evidenced by a certain cartoon sailor's superhuman acts of heroism, spinach is one of the most nutrient-dense foods available. It helps fight cancer with its high levels of antioxidants, heart disease with its vitamin C and beta carotene, and anemia with its excellent iron content.

Besides the veggies used in the following recipes, you can choose from many other options. Try cabbage, mushrooms, cucumbers, squash, zucchini, and all types of peppers, whether eaten by themselves or included in a recipe.

Many people consume white potatoes and corn as their primary vegetables, but they are both foods to be limited on a wheat-free diet. Both spike blood sugar levels.

 We know how tempted you may be to throw a bag of frozen peas into the microwave and call it a side dish, especially at the end of a long day. But by taking a few extra minutes, you can produce a balanced side dish that your family will want seconds of.

Converting veggie-haters into veggie-lovers

One of the tenets of a healthy diet is a heavy emphasis on non-starchy vegetables such as the ones mentioned throughout this book. People sometimes associate a grain-free, low-sugar lifestyle with a diet heavy in meat. That's a mistaken belief. In fact, you'll probably find yourself eating more vegetables than you did before you made the switch. For some, this thought is very unappetizing. If you or a family member feels this way, don't fret. You can overcome your distaste for vegetables.

Several factors are at play when making vegetables desirable:

✔ **Quality:** Choose fresh, organic vegetables whenever possible. You'll be amazed at the taste difference between a typical head of broccoli sold at mass grocers, for example, and a locally grown, organic one. Even the most veggie-averse individual will have to admit the difference and start including them in their meals. Unfortunately, many people grew up thinking vegetables were soggy, mushy substances that came from cans. Understandably, the memory of that taste can be hard to shed. So even if you can't purchase locally grown organic vegetables, fresh ones usually taste better than canned or frozen varieties. (In Mom's defense, fresh produce wasn't as readily available in the olden days as it is today.)

✔ **Changes in taste buds:** As you remove grains and added sugar from your diet, you'll notice subtle changes in how food tastes. The most obvious will be how sweet foods seem. Fruit takes on a whole new dimension, for instance. But, surprisingly, all other foods will make a slide to the sweet side, so to speak. Foods that previously tasted bitter aren't so bitter anymore, including veggies.

✔ **Preparation:** What's old is new again in grain-free, low-sugar eating. Vilified fats like grass-fed butter and bacon grease can and should be part of your kitchen inventory. Adults and kids alike will be more inclined to chow down when veggies are cooked with these tasty and satisfying fats. The recipes in this book use these fats and oils so the whole family can eat together.

The bottom line: If the people you're cooking for are willing to try a new or "yucky" vegetable, don't be surprised when they're satisfied with the taste. You can change the quality of the food you buy and how you prepare it today. However, allow more time for the taste buds to change. It won't happen overnight, but it will happen.

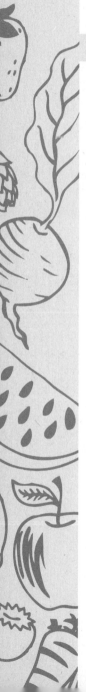

Prosciutto-Wrapped Asparagus and Goat Cheese

Prep time: 10 min • **Cook time:** 1½ min • **Yield:** 4–6 servings

Ingredients	Directions
5 teaspoons salt **1 pound asparagus, tough ends trimmed** **8 thin slices prosciutto** **14-ounce log goat cheese, cut into 24 chunks**	*1* Bring 6 quarts of water to a boil in a large pot over high heat and season with the salt. Cook the asparagus 1 to 1½ minutes until crisp but tender.
	2 Transfer the blanched asparagus to a bowl of ice water and allow to soak until completely cool, about 1 minute. Place atop several layers of paper towels and pat dry.
	3 Cut the prosciutto slices into three pieces. Put one chunk of goat cheese on one end of a prosciutto slice and top with 3 stalks of asparagus.
	4 Roll up the prosciutto bundle, secure it with a toothpick, and set it on a platter. Repeat Steps 3 and 4 with the remaining ingredients and serve.

Per serving: *Calories 89 (From Fat 45); Fat 5g (Saturated 3g); Cholesterol 17mg; Sodium 2,340mg; Carbohydrate 3g (Dietary Fiber 2g); Protein 9g.*

Note: These bundles keep at room temperature for up to 1 hour before serving.

Broccoli and Cheese Casserole

Prep time: 15 min • **Cook time:** 15 min • **Yield:** 6–8 servings

Ingredients	*Directions*
2 pounds broccoli	*1* Preheat the oven to 400 degrees with the rack in the middle position. Trim the florets from the broccoli heads and chop the stalks. Steam the broccoli until it's bright green and crisp but tender, about 5 to 6 minutes. Drain and set aside.
3 tablespoons unsalted butter	
1 medium clove garlic	
½ teaspoon dry mustard	
Pinch cayenne pepper	*2* Melt the butter in a medium saucepan over medium heat. Stir in the garlic, mustard, and cayenne and cook for about 30 seconds. Add the almond flour and cook, stirring constantly, for about 1 minute.
3 tablespoons almond flour	
1½ cups whole milk	
1 cup low-sodium chicken broth	*3* Slowly whisk in the milk and broth. Bring to a simmer and cook, whisking often, for about 5 minutes. Remove the pan from the heat and whisk in the cheeses. Salt and pepper to taste.
8 ounces colby cheese, shredded (about 1⅓ cups)	
4 ounces sharp cheddar cheese, shredded (about 1⅓ cups)	*4* Spray a 13-x-9-inch baking dish with nonstick spray and add the broccoli. Whisk the cheese sauce again and pour it over the broccoli. Bake until golden brown and bubbling around the edges, about 15 minutes.
Salt and pepper to taste	

Per serving: Calories 289 (From Fat 189); Fat 21g (Saturated 12g); Cholesterol 58mg; Sodium 472mg; Carbohydrate 12g (Dietary Fiber 3g); Protein 16g.

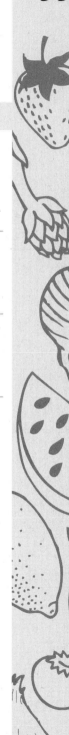

Shaved Brussels Sprouts Salad

Prep time: 5 min • **Cook time:** 5 min • **Yield:** 6 servings

Ingredients	Directions
1½ pounds Brussels sprouts	**1** Very thinly slice the Brussels sprouts with the slicing blade of a food processor and toss them into a bowl.
2 cups walnuts	
⅓ cup finely grated pecorino Romano cheese	**2** Heat a frying pan over medium-high heat. Toast the walnuts in the hot, dry pan for about 5 minutes, stirring frequently so they don't burn. Remove the pan from heat when the nuts start to brown and smell toasted. Remove the nuts from the pan to prevent over-toasting and let them cool.
¼ cup extra-virgin olive oil	
Juice of 1 lemon	
Pepper to taste (optional)	
	3 When the walnuts are cool to the touch, lightly crush them with your hands. Add the walnuts, cheese, oil, and lemon juice to the Brussels sprouts and toss to combine. Season with pepper to taste (if desired).

Per serving: Calories 400 (From Fat 324); Fat 36g (Saturated 4g); Cholesterol 4mg; Sodium 77mg; Carbohydrate 16g (Dietary Fiber 7g); Protein 11g.

Note: You can toast the walnuts a day ahead; keep them in an airtight container at room temperature. You can also preslice the Brussels sprouts up to 3 hours ahead and keep them covered in the refrigerator.

Roasted Cauliflower

Prep time: 10 min • **Cook time:** 25–35 min • **Yield:** 6–8 servings

Ingredients	Directions
1 head of cauliflower (about 2 pounds) **2 tablespoons extra-virgin olive oil** **⅛ teaspoon salt**	**1** Preheat the oven to 450 degrees with the rack on the middle level. Remove the leaves from the cauliflower. Remove the tough stem and cut the cauliflower into florets about 2 inches wide.
	2 Put the florets in a large bowl. Pour the oil over the pieces and add the salt. Toss to coat.
	3 Place the florets on a rimmed baking sheet lined with foil. Cover the baking sheet tightly with foil and cook for 10 to 12 minutes. Remove the foil cover and continue to cook, flipping once, until the cauliflower starts to become golden brown, about 15 to 20 minutes.

Per serving: Calories 58 (From Fat 36); Fat 4g (Saturated 0.5g); Cholesterol 0mg; Sodium 72mg; Carbohydrate 6g (Dietary Fiber 2g); Protein 2g.

Tip: To easily break the cauliflower into florets, cut the head of the cauliflower into two equal wedges and then cut those in half again. Remove the tough stem from each section and cut the wedges into florets.

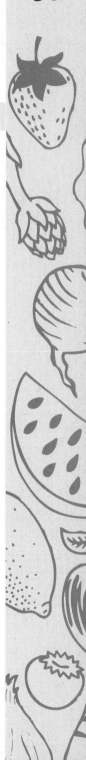

Slow Cooker Collard Greens

Prep time: 6 min • **Cook time:** 5–7 hr • **Yield:** 6–8 servings

Ingredients	Directions
1 onion, peeled and minced	**1** Microwave the onion, garlic, oil, and red pepper flakes in a bowl, stirring occasionally, until the onion is softened, about 5 minutes. Transfer to a slow cooker.
6 cloves garlic, minced	
1 tablespoon avocado oil	
½ teaspoon red pepper flakes	**2** Stir in the collard greens (with stems), the broth, 2 cups of water, the salt, and the vinegar. Submerge the ham hock; cover and cook on low until the collard greens are tender, about 5 to 7 hours.
2 pounds collard greens, stems and leaves cut into 1-inch pieces	
4 cups low-sodium chicken broth	**3** Discard the ham hock. Add the prosciutto and season with pepper and butter to taste.
1 teaspoon salt, plus more to taste	
2 tablespoons apple cider vinegar	
1 smoked ham hock, rinsed	
3 ounces diced prosciutto	
Pepper to taste	
Butter to taste	

Per serving: Calories 139 (From Fat 45); Fat 5g (Saturated 1.5g); Cholesterol 20mg; Sodium 641mg; Carbohydrate 12g (Dietary Fiber 2g); Protein 8g.

Tip: You can keep this dish on the slow cooker's warm setting for 1 to 2 hours before serving.

Note: This dish can be served as a side of greens or as a soup with a vitamin-rich broth.

Kale with Pine Nuts and Currants

Prep time: 5 min • **Cook time:** 10–15 min • **Yield:** 6-8 servings

Ingredients	Directions
2 pounds kale	**1** Separate the leaves of the kale from the stems. Cut the stems into ¼-inch slices and the leaves into 1-inch slices.
2 tablespoons avocado oil	
2 tablespoons butter	
1½ teaspoon kosher salt	**2** Heat the avocado oil and butter in a 12-inch frying pan over medium heat until shimmering. Add the kale stems and sprinkle with half the salt. Sauté for 5 minutes or until softened. Add the pine nuts and currants and toss.
¼ cup toasted pine nuts	
¼ cup currants	
1 teaspoon balsamic vinegar	
	3 Add the kale leaves to the pan, sprinkle with the remaining salt, and toss to combine. Add ¼ cup of water, cover the pan, and cook for 5 minutes until the leaves are tender.
	4 Remove the lid. Toss with the balsamic vinegar to combine. Remove to a platter and serve.

Per serving: Calories 143 (From Fat 90); Fat 10g (Saturated 2.5g); Cholesterol 8mg; Sodium 413mg; Carbohydrate 11g (Dietary Fiber 3g); Protein 6g.

Vary It! You can also use Swiss chard in place of kale and raisins in place of currants.

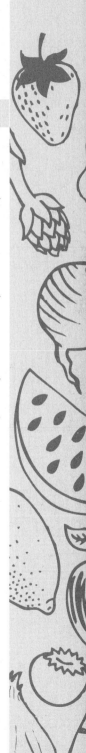

Spinach Salad with Warm Bacon Dressing

Prep time: 20 min • **Cook time:** 20 min • **Yield:** About 6 servings

Ingredients	Directions
3 eggs	*1* Cover the eggs in water in a pot. Bring it to a boil; turn off the heat and let the pot sit for 12 to 14 minutes. Drain and add ice and water to the eggs to speed the cooling.
7 slices thick-cut peppered bacon	
1 small red onion, thinly sliced	*2* Fry the bacon to your desired doneness and remove it to a paper towel. Set aside half of the bacon grease and heat the other half of the grease in a separate skillet over medium heat.
One 8-ounce package white button mushrooms, sliced	
3 tablespoons red wine vinegar	*3* Add the onions to the bacon grease in the second skillet and cook until they're caramelized. Remove to a plate and set aside. Caramelize the mushrooms in the same pan and set aside.
½ teaspoon Dijon mustard	
Dash salt	*4* Chop the bacon. Peel and slice the eggs. Set aside.
8 ounces baby spinach, washed, dried, and stems removed	
	5 In a small saucepan over medium-low heat, whisk together the remaining bacon grease, vinegar, and Dijon mustard. Heat thoroughly.
	6 Put the spinach in a large bowl and top with the onions, mushrooms, and bacon. Pour the hot dressing over the top and toss. Arrange the eggs over the top and serve.

Per serving: Calories 115 (From Fat 63); Fat 7g (Saturated 2g); Cholesterol 104mg; Sodium 283mg; Carbohydrate 5g (Dietary Fiber 2g); Protein 9g.

Chapter 12

Appetizers, Snacks, and Dips

In This Chapter

▶ Having wheat-free snacks at the ready

▶ Enjoying simple offerings for entertaining or snacking

Recipes in This Chapter

↻ Goat Cheese with Bell Pepper Dressing

↻ Baba Gannoujh

↻ Pico de Gallo

▶ Baked Buffalo Wings with Blue Cheese Dip and Veggies

▶ Pepperoni Pizza Snacks

▶ Jalapeños in a Bacon Blanket

*E*veryone has stressed over what to prepare as an appetizer for an upcoming dinner party. Your commitment to a wheat-free lifestyle only adds to the stress because you're not sure whether your guests will enjoy your new diet selections. Fear not! This situation is a great opportunity to spread the wheat-free, low-glycemic message to friends and family. By making the delicious guilt-free recipes in this chapter, you can show your guests they don't have to sacrifice flavor when they say goodbye to wheat. The next thing you know, they'll be begging you for the recipe.

These quick and simple recipes can be served as impressive appetizers or yummy snacks. And you can't beat the convenience of their preparation and clean-up times, either. This is sure to accommodate your family's busy schedule.

The most attractive part of these recipes has to be the ingredient lists. They all include ingredients that are naturally wheat-free. That means no added starch with the removal of gluten. This will keep blood sugar and insulin levels stable, further extending your quest for good health.

Most households struggle to find foods that everyone can agree on. That's not the case with these recipes. You can serve these recipes to a wide audience, thanks to the dishes' diverse range of flavors and textures. From goat cheese to bacon, your entire family is sure to find something to enjoy.

Ready-to-Eat Snacks to Keep on Hand

When you follow a grain-free, low-sugar diet, your blood sugar levels stabilize, which alleviates the need to eat every few hours. When you don't always feel hungry, food won't be on the forefront of your mind. However, sometimes you may want a snack on the go.

For snacks that can be stashed anywhere, make your own granola by mixing some nuts, seeds, shaved unsweetened coconut, and a few raisins. You can also pack a whole avocado with a plastic knife for cutting or take along a couple of dark chocolate squares (at least 70 percent cacao) for a sweet treat.

Some other snacks that are easy to prepare and eat include hard-boiled eggs or a cup of mixed berries. Also try rolling up some meat and cheese from the grocery deli department. Buy each cut a little thicker so they hold their shape for easier handling. And if you want to take any of these snacks with you, buy an insulated bag and an ice pack that will keep food cold and fresh while you're out and about.

Rob's testimonial: Lose the wheat, lose the weight

Saying a cruise changed my life sounds like the beginning of a TV infomercial, but in my case it's the truth. It wasn't so much the cruise itself as the friend I made. For years, I had struggled with my weight. I had high blood pressure and cholesterol that left me taking statins for as long as I can remember. Having tried every diet out there, I had resigned myself to a life of medication and stretchy pants. That was, until Alan started telling me about the benefits of a wheat-free diet.

As soon as the cruise was over, I started to put what I had learned into practice with the hopes of losing some of the weight I gained on the cruise. I jumped in with both feet and began by eliminating wheat from my diet altogether, along with as much sugar and processed oil as possible. Within a week, I started noticing results; not only did the weight start falling off, but I also noticed that I felt better. After a month, I had more energy than I've ever had and was losing weight so consistently that I stopped worrying about weighing and just enjoyed being active.

What shocked me the most was that my reliance on antacids nearly disappeared, as did my sinus issues. Aside from some seasonal allergies, I rarely have sinus issues anymore, and the constant congestion is gone.

I've lost almost 40 pounds and feel better than I've ever felt. I still occasionally eat things I shouldn't, but those indulgences are rare, and I don't crave them anymore. Too much backsliding makes me feel bloated and lethargic and typically sends me straight back to the antacids. Simply avoiding the standard wheat-containing foods works for me. I don't sweat the little things like the occasional sauce with a wheat ingredient or cross-contamination. I only wish I'd given up wheat sooner.

Goat Cheese with Bell Pepper Dressing

Prep time: 10 min, plus standing time • **Cook time:** 8–10 min • **Yield:** 8 servings

Ingredients	Directions
8 tablespoons extra-virgin olive oil, divided	*1* Heat 2 tablespoons of the oil in a medium skillet over medium heat. Add the bell peppers and sauté until they're tender, about 5 minutes.
½ cup diced green bell pepper	
½ cup diced red bell pepper	*2* Reduce the heat to medium-low. Add the garlic, rosemary, coriander, fennel, pepper, thyme, bay leaf, and remaining oil. Simmer for 5 minutes and remove from the heat. Season to taste with salt and let cool to room temperature.
½ cup diced yellow bell pepper	
8 large cloves garlic, thinly sliced	
4 teaspoons chopped fresh rosemary	*3* Arrange the goat cheese slices on a platter and spoon the pepper dressing over them. Let stand for 1 hour at room temperature. Sprinkle with the pine nuts and serve with veggies for dipping.
1 teaspoon coriander seeds, crushed	
½ teaspoon fennel seeds, crushed	
½ teaspoon pepper	
½ teaspoon dried thyme	
1 bay leaf	
Salt to taste	
Two 8-ounce logs goat cheese, cut into 16 slices	
3 tablespoons toasted pine nuts	

Per serving: Calories 305 (From Fat 252); Fat 28g (Saturated 10g); Cholesterol 26mg; Sodium 211mg; Carbohydrate 3g (Dietary Fiber 1g); Protein 11g.

Note: You can also serve this dressing with crackers, but remember to use wheat-free crackers. You can usually find high-fiber crackers made with lots of nuts and seeds that don't have wheat.

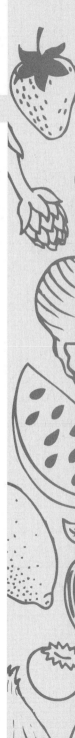

Baba Gannoujh

Prep time: 10 min • **Cook time:** 45 min • **Yield:** 8–10 servings

Ingredients	Directions
2 pounds eggplant	**1** Place an oven rack in the middle position and preheat the oven to 500 degrees.
1 medium clove garlic, minced	
¾ teaspoon salt	**2** Cover a baking sheet with parchment paper. Cut the eggplant(s) in half lengthwise and jab the insides a few times with a fork. Place the eggplant on the baking sheet.
Pinch of cayenne pepper	
3 tablespoons fresh lemon juice	**3** Roast the eggplant for about 45 minutes until it's soft.
¼ cup tahini	
¼ cup extra-virgin olive oil, plus more for garnish	**4** While the eggplant is cooking, combine the garlic, salt, cayenne, lemon juice, tahini, olive oil, and yogurt in a food processor.
¼ cup plain yogurt	
1 teaspoon sesame seeds	**5** After the eggplant is cool enough to handle, scoop out the pulp and drain it in a colander for 3 to 4 minutes. Put the drained pulp in the food processor and blend until smooth.
	6 Pour the eggplant mixture into a bowl and garnish with olive oil and the sesame seeds. Serve with raw veggies.

Per serving: Calories 112 (From Fat 81); Fat 9g (Saturated 1g); Cholesterol 0mg; Sodium 241mg; Carbohydrate 7g (Dietary Fiber 3g); Protein 2g.

Tip: You can make this dip ahead of time and chill it in the refrigerator until you're ready to serve it.

Pico de Gallo

Prep time: 5 min • **Yield:** 4–6 servings

Ingredients	Directions
4 ripe tomatoes or 8 ripe roma tomatoes, cored and diced	**1** Gently mix the tomatoes, onions, jalapeños, lime juice, and cilantro in a glass or stainless steel bowl.
1 cup finely diced sweet yellow onion	
1 large jalapeño, stemmed, seeded, and finely diced	**2** Add 1 teaspoon of salt; mix and taste. If the mixture needs more flavor, add more salt in small increments. Serve or store covered and chilled for up to 2 days.
¼ cup fresh lime juice	
½ cup chopped fresh cilantro	
1 teaspoon salt, plus more to taste	

Per serving: Calories 37 (From Fat 18); Fat 2g (Saturated 0g); Cholesterol 0mg; Sodium 394mg; Carbohydrate 5g (Dietary Fiber 1g); Protein 1g.

Tip: If you like more heat in your pico, use 2 jalapeños.

Note: You can use this salsa to top off Chicken Mexican Soup. Find the recipe in Chapter 10.

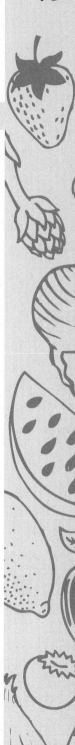

Baked Buffalo Wings with Blue Cheese Dip and Veggies

Prep time: 10 min • **Cook time:** 50 min • **Yield:** About 20 wings

Ingredients	Directions
5 tablespoons butter, divided	*1* Preheat the oven to 450 degrees. Grease a baking sheet with 1 tablespoon of the butter. Scatter the wings on the sheet; bake for 22 to 25 minutes until they're browned. Flip and bake for another 22 to 25 minutes until crispy.
2 pounds frozen chicken wings	
½ cup hot sauce	
½ cup crumbled blue cheese	
3 tablespoons buttermilk	*2* While the wings are baking, warm the hot sauce and remaining butter in a saucepan on low for 5 minutes and then remove it from the heat.
3 tablespoons sour cream	
2 teaspoons white wine vinegar	*3* Mash the blue cheese and buttermilk in a small bowl with a fork. Stir in the sour cream and vinegar.
4 carrots, cut into 2-inch sticks	
4 celery stalks, cut into 2-inch sticks	*4* Put the crispy wings and the sauce in a large bowl and stir until the wings are coated. (If all the wings won't fit in the bowl at once, mix them in batches.) Serve them immediately with the carrots, celery sticks, and blue cheese dip on the side.

Per serving: Calories 148 (From Fat 99); Fat 11g (Saturated 3.5g); Cholesterol 46mg; Sodium 348mg; Carbohydrate 2g (Dietary Fiber 0.5g); Protein 9g.

Note: The wings must be crispy when they go into the sauce, or the sauce will slide right off. You can get crispier wings by patting them dry before you bake them. The sauce will keep for 1 week in the fridge, and the blue cheese dip will keep for about 4 days.

Vary It! The recipe as written makes mild to medium sauce. For a truly hot sauce, just use the hot sauce (we like Frank's Louisiana Hot Sauce) with no butter added.

Pepperoni Pizza Snacks

Prep time: 5 min • **Cook time:** 15 min • **Yield:** 4 servings

Ingredients	Directions
5 to 7 ounces large pepperoni slices (about 20 to 30 pieces) 4 ounces marinara sauce 4 ounces grated mozzarella cheese	**1** Preheat the oven to 400 degrees. Bake the pepperoni on a baking sheet covered with parchment paper for 8 minutes, flipping once.
	2 Remove the baking sheet from the oven. Divide the marinara evenly among the pepperonis and top with the cheese. Bake for 5 more minutes.

Per serving: Calories 346 (From Fat 261); Fat 29g (Saturated 12g); Cholesterol 68mg; Sodium 1,199mg; Carbohydrate 4g (Dietary Fiber 0.5g); Protein 17g.

Tip: The first 8 minutes of baking are crucial if you want the pepperonis to be crispy.

Vary It! You can dice your favorite pizza vegetable toppings and add them as well before the final 5 minutes of bake time.

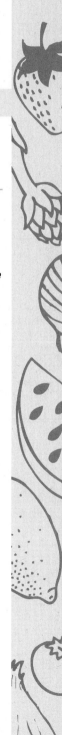

Jalapeños in a Bacon Blanket

Prep time: 20 min • **Cook time:** 20–25 min • **Yield:** 10 servings

Ingredients	Directions
20 whole fresh 2-to-3-inch jalapeños 4 ounces softened cream cheese 1 pound sliced bacon, cut into thirds	*1* Preheat the oven to 375 degrees. Wearing gloves, cut the jalapeños in half lengthwise and scoop out the seeds and white membranes.
	2 Smear the cream cheese into the jalapeño boats and wrap each with a piece of bacon, securing with a toothpick through the middle.
	3 Bake on a pan with a wire rack for 20 minutes. If the bacon isn't brown enough, turn the broiler on for a few minutes. Serve hot or at room temperature.

Per serving: Calories 292 (From Fat 207); Fat 23g (Saturated 8g); Cholesterol 62mg; Sodium 1,085mg; Carbohydrate 3g (Dietary Fiber 1g); Protein 18g.

Tip: Don't let the bacon shrink so much that it squeezes the jalapeño. If the bacon shrinks too much, the cream cheese may ooze out.

Tip: You may want to wear some latex gloves while prepping the jalapeño so you don't get the heat-causing substances on your hands (and then perhaps in your eyes). Figure 12-1 shows you how to seed a jalapeño.

Figure 12-1:
How to seed a jalapeño pepper without getting burned.

Seeding a Jalapeño

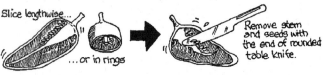

Slice lengthwise...

...or in rings

Remove stem and seeds with the end of rounded table knife.

CAREFUL!
Some say use rubber gloves or dip fingers in lemon juice and use lots of soap and water!

Illustration by Elizabeth Kurtzman

Chapter 13

Baked Goods Like You Never Thought Possible

For most people, the idea of giving up eating baked goods, whether packaged or homemade, is very difficult. If you aren't a sweets eater, you can skip to the next chapter. However, if you're used to something sweet after every meal, then a low-glycemic, wheat-free diet may pose a challenge. With a little knowledge of the right ingredient replacements, though, yummy foods are yours for the baking.

Our recommendation, as always, is to go cold turkey with wheat, sugar, and alternative sweeteners; this strategy is the best way to change your tastes and diminish your desire for sweet foods. You won't believe how sweet plain fruit will taste! When you've reset your taste buds, you'll need less (or no) alternative sweetener.

In this chapter, we give you the lowdown on the best wheat-free flour options and the two most common replacement sweeteners (sugar substitutes and sugar alcohols). Be sure to check out the recipes for goodies in this chapter as well!

Considering Wheat-Free Flour Alternatives

Alternatives to wheat-based flour are easier to find today in specialty and even average grocery stores than they were a couple of years ago. If you can't find them where you shop, ask the store manager whether he can order the flour for you, or go online to purchase them.

Here are our four favorites:

- **Almond flour:** You can buy almond flour already ground or do it yourself. Use sprouted almonds and a blender or food processor, and you're good to go. Regular whole almonds will suffice, but we recommend the sprouted variety because the sprouting process destroys most of the enzyme inhibitors, allowing for better digestion and more nutrient availability.

- **Buckwheat flour:** Easily obtained in better grocery stores, buckwheat flour, harvested from a seed, is high in magnesium, fiber, and protein.

- **Coconut flour:** Coconut flour is a very healthy alternative, though it does require a bit more liquid because it absorbs a lot of moisture. Use an egg for every ¼ cup of coconut flour to add moisture and to help the flour bind to other ingredients. We also recommend combining coconut flour with another flour; if you don't, you may find the coconut flavor overwhelming.

- **Flaxmeal:** Flax is another healthy alternative; it's popular among vegetarians, who use it as one of the few sources of omega-3 fatty acids in their diets. Flax is best absorbed in meal (ground) form, not as the whole seeds.

Buy a cheap coffee grinder and use it solely for grinding flax and the like. Using it for coffee will leave a permanent coffee odor and result in flax that tastes like coffee.

One of the first rules with using alternative flours is to replace the amounts by weight, not by volume. For example, ¼ cup of refined flour is 2 ounces; you want to measure out 2 ounces of the replacement, not ¼ cup. The exception is buckwheat flour; you can substitute this flour for refined flour with the exact volume required. No need to weigh it.

Seeking Sugar Alternatives

When you rid your diet of added sugar and alternative sweeteners, you take another step toward preventing the damage that high blood glucose levels can lead to.

Although we highly recommend going cold turkey with all things sweet, many people find this to be the most difficult change that a wheat-free diet requires. However, you can turn to sugar alternatives that have few to no negative effects on the body. You just need to limit the treats containing these acceptable alternatives so you can reduce the craving signals the brain generates.

Picking the right sugar substitute

Notice we didn't say the right sugar substitutes, plural. There's really only one thing you can use in place of refined white sugar, and that's stevia. *Stevia* is a plant grown in South America. It doesn't raise insulin levels and is nearly 300 times sweeter than sugar, which is why you need to use only a tiny droplet of it for most recipes.

Buy stevia in as close to a 100-percent extract as possible. Like many products that are mass-produced, this sweetener can come in a highly processed form, which you should avoid because of the chemicals used in the processing.

For our recipes, we use spoonable Stevita. Because stevia is so sweet, it's sometimes difficult to bake with. Stevita is mixed with erythritol (a sugar alcohol we describe in the following section), so 1 teaspoon equals 3 teaspoons of sugar. You can buy Stevita in a jar or in individual packets.

We don't recommend artificial sweeteners (the kinds you see in any mass-produced food or drink with the words *no-calorie* or *zero-calories* on the label). The most popular, aspartame (found in NutraSweet and Equal), accounts for the most negative reactions of any food additive, including headaches, mood swings, seizures, neurological disorders, and emotional and behavioral disorders. Other popular alternatives include sucralose (Splenda), a highly processed substance containing chlorine, and saccharin (Sweet'N Low), a possible cause of cancer.

Baking with sugar alcohols

Sugar alcohols are a hybrid carbohydrate that somewhat resemble sugar and somewhat resemble alcohol. (That's why the name makes sense.) They occur naturally in plants. Because they aren't completely absorbed by the body, they don't have a major impact on blood sugar levels.

The flip side to sugar alcohols not being completely absorbed is that they can cause bloating, gas, or possibly diarrhea. Everyone responds differently, so don't go overboard with sugar alcohols until you know how well you tolerate them. Increased use will also increase tolerance.

The most common sugar alcohols are xylitol, sorbitol, maltitol, and erythritol. Xylitol and sorbitol are common in items such as gum and ice cream but not so much in baking. Maltitol is used in baked goods, but we don't recommend it because of its tendency to raise blood sugar. Which brings us to erythritol, the best of the sugar alcohols, especially for baking. It causes the least gastrointestinal distress, doesn't affect blood sugar, and won't cause cavities.

Erythritol is sold in crystal and powder form and is generally labeled "erythritol."

Larry's story: Experiment leads to a better life

Like most everyone around me, I thought my constant hunger, weight gain, frequent heartburn, low energy level, and regular colds were normal. I never really considered that my diet could be responsible for these things. I tried to eat right by following the lowfat, lots-of-whole-grain guidelines that had been recommended for 30 years. And at 49 years old, I thought a lot of my normal was just me getting older.

All that started to change when I read a book that suggested that maybe sugars and refined carbohydrates were the foods I should be concerned with eliminating. Being the scientist I am, I set out to conduct an experiment on myself by radically changing my diet. I cut out all sugars and refined carbs: Bread, cookies, cakes, ice cream, sandwiches — if it was processed, I didn't eat it. I added lots of eggs (yolks and all) and grass-fed meats. I started cooking with real butter and coconut oil. I snacked on nuts, seeds, and avocadoes and continued eating fruits and vegetables.

Completely changing my diet was hard at first. But after the initial withdrawal symptoms subsided, a funny thing happened: I felt better! I had energy — no more 2 p.m. daily naps. I started losing weight, and I wasn't hungry between meals. I continued to see improvement; my body fat dropped to below 10 percent, and my good cholesterol improved. I'm maintaining my weight almost effortlessly and, most importantly, I really enjoy the foods I eat. I'm five years into my experiment, and it's become a lifestyle I can live with.

Cashew Butter and Chocolate Chip Cookies

Prep time: 10 min • **Cook time:** 22 min • **Yield:** About 48 cookies

Ingredients	Directions
4 tablespoons butter	*1* Preheat the oven to 350 degrees with a rack in the center. Cover two cookie sheets with parchment paper.
1 cup almond flour	
1 cup coconut flour	*2* Melt the butter in the microwave for 30 seconds. Let cool. In a small bowl, whisk the almond flour, coconut flour, salt, baking soda, and Stevita.
1 teaspoon salt	
1 teaspoon baking soda	
1 packet Stevita	*3* In a large bowl, mix the eggs, vanilla, almond milk, and melted butter with a hand mixer. Add the cashew butter and mix for 1 minute.
4 eggs	
2 teaspoons sugar-free vanilla	
⅔ cup almond milk	*4* Pour the dry ingredients into the wet ingredients. Mix with a hand mixer. Fold in the chocolate chips by hand.
¾ cup cashew butter	
12 ounces 63% cacao dark chocolate chips	*5* Place 1-tablespoon balls of dough ½ inch apart on the cookie sheets and push down with the back of a spoon to flatten. Bake one pan at a time for 11 minutes.
	6 Let the cookies cool on the sheet for a minute and then remove to a cooling rack.

Per serving: Calories 102 (From Fat 56); Fat 8g (Saturated 3g); Cholesterol 18mg; Sodium 85mg; Carbohydrate 7g (Dietary Fiber 2g); Protein 3g.

Vary It! You can break up a 12-ounce chocolate bar with an even higher cacao percentage instead of using chocolate chips.

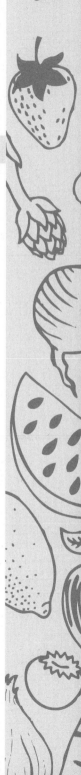

Black Bean Brownies

Prep time: 10 min • **Cook time:** 22–24 min • **Yield:** 12 brownies

Ingredients	Directions
One 15-ounce can black beans, drained and well rinsed	**1** Preheat the oven to 350 degrees. Lightly grease a 12-cup muffin pan.
2 eggs	
4 tablespoons butter, melted and cooled	**2** Puree all the ingredients in a food processor for about 3 minutes, scraping down the sides as needed.
¾ cup high-quality cocoa powder	
1 teaspoon sea salt	**3** Divide the batter equally into the muffin pan. Bake for 22 to 24 minutes or until the edges start to pull away from the sides. Remove from the oven and let cool before removing from pan.
1 teaspoon sugar-free vanilla extract	
¼ cup honey	
1 teaspoon Stevita	
1 teaspoon baking powder	
2 teaspoons espresso, liquid or powdered	

Per serving: Calories 108 (From Fat 54); Fat 6g (Saturated 3g); Cholesterol 41mg; Sodium 298mg; Carbohydrate 14g (Dietary Fiber 3g); Protein 4g.

Vary It! You can also add walnuts, pecans, or dark chocolate chips to the tops of the muffins before you put them in the oven.

Swapping beans for flour in baked goods

The first and only rule of swapping beans for flour when baking is don't tell the person eating the goodie what's in the recipe! When someone does ask, "What's your secret?" after enjoying a black bean brownie, for instance, tell him and then watch the look on his face when he realizes you actually said "black beans."

The substitution is easy: one 15-ounce can of black beans for 1 cup of flour. The substitution reduces the calorie content and increases protein and fiber content, all without changing the texture of the final product. You can use white or navy beans in recipes that require a lighter color, such as chocolate chip cookies.

Cinnamon Coffee Cake

Prep time: 15 min • **Cook time:** 45 min, plus cooling time • **Yield:** 10 servings

Ingredients	Directions
2 cups almond flour	**1** Preheat the oven to 325 degrees and grease a Bundt pan with butter. In a medium bowl, whisk the almond flour, buckwheat flour, whey protein, baking powder, baking soda, salt, and 2 tablespoons of erythritol.
1 cup buckwheat flour	
¼ cup unflavored whey protein	
1 teaspoon baking powder	**2** In a separate medium bowl, mix the sour cream and eggs with a mixer until smooth. Scrape down the sides and add the butter. Beat for one minute on medium speed. Beat in the flour mixture.
1 teaspoon baking soda	
1 teaspoon salt	
½ cup plus 5 tablespoons erythritol, divided	**3** Pour half of the mixture into the pan and smooth the top. Combine the cinnamon, ½ cup of erythritol, and 20 drops of stevia; sprinkle the mixture over the batter in the pan. Spread the remaining batter over the top and smooth.
1 cup sour cream	
3 eggs	
4 tablespoons melted butter, cooled	**4** Bake for 45 minutes; let cool in the pan for 15 minutes. Flip out onto a wire rack and let cool completely.
2 teaspoons ground cinnamon	
20 drops stevia	**5** In a small bowl, beat the cream cheese, 3 tablespoons of erythritol, cream, and vanilla. Drizzle over the cooled cake.
3 tablespoons softened cream cheese	
1 tablespoon heavy whipping cream	
½ teaspoon vanilla extract	

Per serving: Calories 312 (From Fat 216); Fat 24g (Saturated 8g); Cholesterol 98mg; Sodium 445mg; Carbohydrate 30g (Dietary Fiber 4g); Protein 14g.

Part IV

Embracing the Wheat-Free Lifestyle

Code Words that Wheat May Hide Behind

Battered	Breaded
Coated	Creamy
Crispy	Croutons
Crumbs	Crunchy
Crusted	Encrusted
Fried or deep fried	Grated (cheese)
Marinade	Parmesan (as in chicken parmesan)
Soufflé	Seasonings

Sometimes when you're traveling, you may want to order room service. For tips on making sure you get a wheat-free meal, check out the free article at www.dummies. com/extras/livingwheatfree.

In this part...

- Dining out or traveling can present challenges to maintaining your wheat- or grain-free lifestyle. Get some tips to make navigating these situations easier.

- Discover how to enjoy get-togethers with family and friends while sticking to your wheat/grain-free diet. Be a good wheat-free ambassador by deftly handling questions and comments about your choices.

- Any lifestyle with optimal health as a goal requires exercise as a major component. Check out more than a dozen exercises to get you started.

- Lab tests can confirm what your body is already telling you: You're getting healthier. See which medical tests we recommend to evaluate your health.

- Regardless of how nutritional your wheat- or grain-free diet is, you may need additional supplements to maintain or improve your health. Check out the list of essential nutrients to make sure you're getting enough of them.

Chapter 14

Dining Out around Town and While Traveling

In This Chapter

▶ Selecting a restaurant to meet your wheat-free needs

▶ Navigating a restaurant's menu

▶ Planning for wheat-free travel

*A*lthough having a meal out that's all organic, grass-fed, and wild-caught, is prepared without vegetable oil, and contains little or no wheat or sugar (or, ideally, grain of any kind) is next to impossible, you can achieve a couple of these ideals if you do some homework before you head out the door.

After you get the hang of eating wheat-free at various restaurants, dining out is a snap. Becoming familiar with the restaurants in your area, figuring out how to decode the menu, and developing a question/answer dialogue with the restaurant staff helps you determine which restaurants meet your needs.

This chapter is designed to help you build confidence in dining out on a wheat-free diet. We discuss how to best manage a meal when getting the ideal meal isn't possible and highlight restaurant chains that have added gluten-free menus to accommodate folks with a wheat-free way of life. (Though you may not be gluten-free, gluten-free food is inherently wheat-free, as we explain in Chapter 3.) We recommend ways to interpret a typical restaurant menu and provide tips on staying wheat-free while traveling.

For those with celiac disease, the most important thing to remember when dining out is to speak to your server about the severity of your condition. This way, the server can discuss with the chef and coordinate with the kitchen regarding the allergy. Just because a restaurant has a gluten-free menu doesn't mean that cross-contamination won't happen, so although we try to give you the best options for dining out on a wheat-free diet, know that there are no guarantees for those who eat wheat-free because of celiac and severe intolerances.

Choosing the Right Restaurant

It used to be that if you asked for a list of wheat-free or gluten-free items a restaurant served, you'd get a funny look from the waiter and would be told that the restaurant didn't offer those types of meals. Today, identifying wheat-free and gluten-free items on a menu is much easier. Some restaurants even mark them with a special icon.

But first you have to find those restaurants. Always do your homework ahead of time and be proactive in your restaurant search. Online directories actually list restaurants with gluten-free menus. After you find a viable candidate, read the restaurant's website menu or call and talk to the chef or manager to figure out whether the restaurant can meet your needs. If one of your favorite restaurants doesn't offer what you need in wheat-free form, don't be afraid to ask the chef whether she's willing to prepare a wheat-free alternative that you provide. Just make sure you ask ahead of time.

In this section, we list some chain restaurants that can meet your wheat-free needs, and we explain how to find other workable restaurants in your area. We also show you what to look out for when dining at ethnic restaurants and how to navigate fast-food joints if you can't avoid them. Then we help you manage your expectations when dining out.

Restaurants recognize the need for gluten-free dishes

In 2000, you could almost hear a giant sigh of relief from the wheat sufferers around the country. The Gluten-Free Restaurant Awareness Program (GFRAP), operated by the Gluten Intolerance Group, began spreading the gluten-free message to restaurants near and far. Finally, the cry of the wheat-sensitive was being heard!

Restaurants began providing gluten-free menus, and with the new menus came restaurant staff training. GFRAP was revamped in 2013 as the Gluten-Free Food Service Management and Training Program (GFFS). The GFFS certification program ensures that a restaurant has met certain guidelines sufficient to be called gluten-free. So you can be confident that restaurants that are certified gluten-free have well-trained staffs and are equipped to handle your questions and needs.

Other people who have benefitted from the GFFS are those who have to eliminate wheat from their diets for health purposes. These people may not share the same gluten difficulties as those with gluten intolerance or celiac disease, but they are concerned with reducing their inflammation, gastric distress, elevated blood sugar, and allergies. The GFFS has provided a win/win for all involved.

Knowing what to look for

Whether you're perusing a menu online or at the restaurant or calling to speak with the chef, you need some kind of guideline for determining whether an establishment can provide the wheat-free service you need. Here's a checklist of things to seek out when dining out:

- ✓ **A lengthy gluten- or wheat-free menu:** For most people looking out for their wheat consumption, having just a couple of gluten-free items on the menu isn't enough. Nothing is more unpleasant than going to a restaurant where you can't eat any of the food.

- ✓ **A knowledgeable waitstaff:** How much the servers know is a good indicator of how well trained the rest of the employees at the restaurant are.

- ✓ **Ingredients lists that are available to patrons:** What ingredients are in the sauces and salad dressings on the menu? Can you have a list of ingredients for other items (breads, desserts) that may contain wheat?

- ✓ **Fresh, quality food items:** Fresh protein (beef, fish, chicken), fruits and vegetables, beans, and nonprocessed foods are important parts of your wheat-free lifestyle. Not all restaurants have them because of the high cost, but it's well worth the search.

- ✓ **A manager who can discuss the restaurant's food preparation conditions and techniques:** Is the cooking staff knowledgeable on handling food so that cross-contamination with wheat and gluten doesn't occur? This issue is a biggie for celiac patients and highly sensitive wheat and gluten sufferers.

- ✓ **A separate kitchen or cooking area and dishwashing area:** Separate facilities help cut down on careless cross-contamination when people are handling your food.

Finding wheat-free chain restaurants

The search for restaurants with gluten-free menus has become less daunting because awareness of wheat's harmful effects has grown such that even places with measly gluten-free options are promoting their "gluten-free menu." In any case, many restaurants are looking to expand their customer reach, so they're becoming more accommodating to the gluten-free market to remain competitive with other restaurants that are doing the same.

Even chain restaurants offer gluten-free menus. Many of these restaurants don't offer gluten-free kitchens, though, so cross-contamination may be an issue, especially for wheat's most sensitive sufferers. Remember to call ahead to see whether the restaurant meets your satisfaction. And don't assume a menu tagged "gluten-free" means you're off the hook for asking questions about preparation methods and so on; you still have to do some due diligence.

Here are some chains that offer gluten-free menus:

- Austin Grill (Tex-Mex)
- Biaggi's Ristorante Italiano (Italian)
- Boston Market (American)
- Carrabba's Italian Grill (Italian)
- Chili's (American)
- Fleming's Prime Steakhouse and Wine Bar (Steakhouse)
- Olive Garden (Italian)
- On The Border (Mexican)
- Outback Steakhouse (Steakhouse)
- P.F. Chang's China Bistro (Asian)
- Red Lobster (Seafood)
- Red Robin (American)
- Romano's Macaroni Grill (Italian)
- Ruby Tuesday's (American)
- Souper Salad (American)

To find other restaurants in your area that offer wheat-free or gluten-free meals, simply enter the name of your city and "wheat-free restaurant" into your favorite search engine. Chances are, you'll get some decent results, and you can explore from there. You may want to repeat your search every few months because the restaurant landscape changes all the time. You never know which establishments have added wheat- and gluten-free options to their menus.

Enjoying international cuisines

One of life's greatest pleasures is enjoying food from diverse parts of the world. But when dining out in ethnic restaurants, the greatest challenge can be the language barrier, particularly if you need to ask questions of someone who doesn't speak your language. The more wheat sensitive you are, the more you need the restaurant staff to understand your situation. If the language barrier is too great to overcome, we suggest politely leaving and finding a restaurant where you can communicate your needs effectively.

Even though you may be able to eat a wheat-free meal at different ethnic restaurants, that meal may still trigger health effects like insulin spikes. Minimizing sugar and vegetable oil consumption in addition to wheat helps prevent the long-term effects of spiking insulin levels and inflammation.

Here is a list of what to be on the lookout for when you eat at ethnic restaurants:

- ✔ **Chinese:** Steering clear of soy sauce (which contains wheat) is the name of the game with Chinese food because almost every Chinese dish contains it. A chicken or beef stir-fry without the gluten-filled sauces is sure to satisfy.

- ✔ **Greek:** Greek restaurants can be problematic because of the wheat pastas and thickened sauces used in many dishes. Greek menus have a variety of grilled meats you can order with a Greek feta salad. Just watch out for the marinades.

- ✔ **Italian:** With all the pastas, bread, and sauces associated with Italian food, managing a night out in Little Italy can be challenging. When you're looking for a safe wheat-free option, the caprese salad and antipasto appetizer and a grilled lamb, beef, or sausage dish should do the trick.

- ✔ **Japanese:** You can definitely enjoy the gluten-free world of Japanese food if you like sushi. With the exception of food dipped in soy sauce and batter, you should find plenty of wheat-free options available to you, such as grilled fish.

- ✔ **Mexican:** The major offenders of the Mexican cuisine — flour tortillas, chips, and certain sauces — make up a large portion of the Mexican food restaurant experience. Try the fajita salad or fajitas without the tortillas.

- ✔ **Thai:** Thai restaurants offer many wheat-free options, primarily because a lot of Thai food is naturally gluten-free. Be sure to ask whether the soy sauce used is gluten-free. If it's made in-house, it may well be, but if it's a Chinese-style soy sauce, it probably has plenty of gluten. One delicious dish found at Thai restaurants is grilled fish (without the sauce) and vegetables.

Making the best of fast food in a pinch

With the need for speed in today's hustle-and-bustle lifestyle, fast food restaurants are more popular than ever in spite of the widely held belief that the food is unhealthy. To the industry's credit, several restaurants have attempted to create healthier menus. However, the fast food industry still often uses low-quality meat and oils and lots of wheat and sugar in its items.

Not many fast-food restaurants approach their menus with a low-wheat or wheat-free mentality. The few foods deemed gluten-free are typically prepared in unhealthy vegetable oil in non-dedicated frying pans and baskets, which leads to cross-contamination with wheat foods almost every time.

With the exception of a few places (such as Chick-Fil-A, Wendy's, and Arby's), most of these eating establishments are very limited in their wheat-free items. Eating wheat-free at a fast food restaurant is like rowing a boat upstream; it's a whole lot of effort with little return.

You can probably find some items on most fast food restaurant menus that can be altered to the point of being wheat-free, such as salads and bunless hamburgers. In any case, you must ask many questions about how the food is prepared and its gluten-free status. Note, however, that many establishments aren't educated as to what wheat-free/gluten-free really means. Explaining how to alter your food in a way that fits your needs may be difficult and time consuming.

Although settling for fast food isn't the best possible situation to be in, the following fast food restaurants have varying degrees of gluten-free options:

- ✔ Arby's
- ✔ Au Bon Pain
- ✔ Burger King
- ✔ Chick-Fil-A
- ✔ Chipotle
- ✔ Culver's
- ✔ Dairy Queen
- ✔ Domino's Pizza
- ✔ Godfather's Pizza

- ✔ Jason's Deli
- ✔ Jack-in-the-Box
- ✔ Long John Silver's
- ✔ Panera Bread
- ✔ Sonic Drive-In
- ✔ Starbucks (primarily drinks)
- ✔ Subway
- ✔ Wendy's

Aiming for "manageable," not "perfect"

Imagine that you've researched the best restaurants in town that will accommodate your wheat-free lifestyle. Your restaurant of choice offers a gluten-free menu with a separate kitchen area designated just for preparing gluten-free dishes. You're assured that the dishwashing detergent is wheat-free, so you don't have to worry about any wheat film covering your eating utensils. The menu has grass-fed beef, organic chicken, and wild-caught salmon. All the produce is organic. Any oils used to prepare your food come from coconut, avocado, or olive oil. Now that's the perfect meal out!

Sadly, the chances of eating this perfect restaurant meal are virtually nil. Although many restaurants go to great extremes to provide their patrons with the best dining experience possible, maintaining gluten-free standards this rigorous can become too cost-prohibitive.

Unless you have a strong wheat or gluten sensitivity — such as a severe allergy, a digestive problem, or celiac disease — finding a manageable situation is much more realistic. (Flip to Chapter 3 for details on wheat intolerance conditions.) Luckily, most restaurants fall under the category of "manageable." Even though they may lack a gluten-free menu, most restaurants will help you create your own wheat- or grain-free dish. However, these restaurants won't provide you with a dedicated gluten-free cooking environment. You have to make the call as to whether that's okay based on your level of wheat sensitivity and desire for wheat reduction.

If your favorite restaurants don't offer gluten-free menus or won't assist you with eliminating the wheat from your meal, they're way behind the times. We recommend finding a new regular spot; your health is worth it.

Managing the Menu without Prior Research

Even with the best of intentions, you'll inevitably find yourself in a situation where calling the restaurant or looking online ahead of time isn't possible. Knowing what to look for on the menu, what to avoid, and what questions to ask the waitstaff becomes essential. We cover each of those topics in the following sections.

Cracking the code: Menu keywords to avoid

A lot of restaurant menus have . . . creative ways of describing their food. Although some food descriptions are confusing, others can be downright misleading and are giant red flags for wheat-free eaters. Always ask your server, the manager, or a restaurant kitchen employee (we recommend at least two of the three) to disclose *everything* that's in a food you're considering ordering.

As you're taking in the menu, watch for the following terms that are typically code for gluten. You should avoid them unless you can confirm they're gluten-free. (Some of these are cooking techniques that may be used with wheat-free substitutes, such as almond flour, coconut flour, or crushed pecans.)

- ✔ Battered
- ✔ Breaded
- ✔ Coated
- ✔ Creamy
- ✔ Crispy
- ✔ Croutons
- ✔ Crumbs
- ✔ Crunchy
- ✔ Crusted
- ✔ Dusted
- ✔ En Croute

- ✔ Encrusted
- ✔ Fried or deep fried
- ✔ Grated (cheese)
- ✔ Marinade
- ✔ Parmesan (as in chicken parmesan)
- ✔ Raspings
- ✔ Soufflé
- ✔ Seasonings
- ✔ Stroganoff
- ✔ Wellington

If a restaurant doesn't have a gluten-free menu, you may want to order the most basic meal on the menu. Or, see whether the kitchen will create a plate for you with a piece of meat and a vegetable. If you go the create-your-own-plate route, confirm that everything is wheat-free and meets your level of satisfaction. Some restaurants actually do a good job of making the simple meal tasty.

In this day and age, most restaurants can do a good job of providing you with an outstanding wheat-free experience. If you're not satisfied with your meal, chalk it up as another restaurant that can't meet your needs.

Ferreting out more info

Of all the steps you can take to assure you get the wheat-free treatment you deserve from a restaurant, the most important one stems from the conversations that you have with the chef, manager, and waitstaff. These exchanges are your opportunity to see how much the employees know about the preparation and service of wheat-free food.

We recommend asking the following questions when you speak to the chef, manager, or waitstaff at the restaurant. Your conversations may generate new questions as well:

- ✔ Do you have a gluten-free menu?
- ✔ Do you know what gluten-free truly means?
- ✔ What level of gluten- and wheat-free training do you and your staff have?
- ✔ Are you equipped to serve someone with a wheat or gluten sensitivity?

✔ Do you have a separate area where you prepare gluten-free foods?

✔ Do you change your gloves after handling other food?

✔ What steps do you take to make sure that cross-contamination with wheat/gluten doesn't occur?

✔ Can you show me the list of ingredients in the salad dressing, condiment, or sauce I'll be eating?

✔ Would you double-check with the chef to make sure my gluten-free order is gluten-free?

It never hurts to ask. The more questions you ask, the more information you get, and information is crucial when you're avoiding wheat.

Sometimes your questions won't be answered to your satisfaction no matter how many or which ones you ask. When you don't trust the answers you're getting or someone can't answer your questions to your liking, leave and go somewhere else. It's just not worth the risk.

Tackling Wheat-Free Travel

At first, traveling to a foreign place and eating different food in unfamiliar restaurants seems like an impossible task. However, planning ahead can make the impossible possible.

Having a plan in place rather than leaving your meals to chance helps you to stay on track with your wheat-free or grain-free diet. Too many people throw in the towel and say, "When in Rome . . . ," with the intention of resuming their diets after they return home. Your efforts must be intentional. A healthy wheat-free lifestyle doesn't just happen. Use the travel tips in the following sections to help you stay wheat-free.

If you find chain restaurants that work for you, you've overcome a huge obstacle of wheat-free travel. We list some chains with wheat-free offerings in the earlier section "Finding wheat-free chain restaurants."

Traveling with a wheat-free mindset

Traveling brings a welcome change of pace, but it can be stressful at the same time. You leave behind daily routines and familiar locales. Many of your everyday conveniences aren't at your fingertips, so sticking to your wheat-free diet can be difficult.

Vacations tend to promote an attitude of anything's fair game. We often hear, "Well, I'm on vacation and I'll eat whatever I want," or, "One of the reasons I'm going to that part of the world is for its fantastic food." People complain about gaining weight on vacation because they end up blowing their diets. If you're eating wheat-free, sticking to your guns while on vacation can be particularly challenging.

Business trips, on the other hand, don't tend to encourage that caution-to-the-wind mindset as much. Most people are more likely to continue their normal eating habits (good or bad) while away on business, so there's less temptation to go crazy with food choices if you eat well at home.

Going prepared

Whether the nature of your travels is business or leisure, you must consider beforehand how you want to address your dietary needs. A lack of preparation is sure to send your well-intended wheat-free diet reeling. Here are some things to think about when considering your food options for traveling:

- ✔ What's your level of wheat/gluten sensitivity?
- ✔ How important is it to you to stay wheat-free while you're traveling?
- ✔ What's your level of commitment to your wheat-free lifestyle?
- ✔ After your diet plan is in place, what are some obstacles that could interfere with it?
- ✔ What's your plan B if your initial plan fails?
- ✔ How much prep time do you have before leaving on your trip?
- ✔ Are you flying or driving to your destination? What are your food options while on the airplane or in the car?
- ✔ How long will your traveling take?
- ✔ Where's the nearest health food grocery store where you're staying?
- ✔ Are you staying in a hotel, with a friend, in a tent or no-frills cabin, or in a rented house or condo?
  - • If you're staying in a hotel, will you have access to a refrigerator?
  - • If you're staying with friends, how accommodating will they be to your dietary needs?
  - • Will you have access to a kitchen or other cooking equipment?
- ✔ Will the restaurants available at your destination cater to your wheat-free needs?
- ✔ How long will your trip last?

How you answer these questions depends on your level of wheat sensitivity and your commitment to the wheat-free lifestyle. If you have celiac disease (can't tolerate gluten) or are highly sensitive to wheat or other grains, you must plan your food intake very carefully. If you have some flexibility with how you eat, your trip may be a little easier to manage. However, remember that tightening up your diet when you return home is much more difficult than simply sticking to it on your trip.

The following tips include options for easier access to wheat-free foods when you're traveling. They can help prevent you from getting stuck without a wheat-free option:

✔ If you're traveling on business, identify where your meals will take place before you set sail. Will they be on your own in restaurants or in a hotel, or will they come in the form of buffets and sit-down dinners at a conference? If the food is being provided for you, contact the person in charge of food planning to make sure she's aware of your wheat-free needs. Make sure you have plenty of wheat-free snacks available in case of an emergency.

✔ If you're going camping or staying in a rented condo/house, take your own food. Include whole food items such as eggs, proteins, fruits, and vegetables. You'll have 100 percent control over what you're eating. You may want to take your own eating utensils as well if you're not sure what will be provided for you; that also helps eliminate any chance for cross-contamination.

✔ If you're staying in a hotel, you may also be able to bring a lot of your own food. Call the hotel to determine whether your room will have a refrigerator and/or whether any cooking facilities will be available to you. If a fridge isn't available, stick to non-refrigerated items.

✔ If you're flying, eat a low-carbohydrate meal prior to take off so that you're less likely to become hungry during the flight. Pack snacks such as nuts and seeds in your carry-on and stash several small bags of snacks within your larger bag so you can have snacks throughout your trip. Depending on your destination, you may be able to bring a small cooler as a carry-on. In that case, you can pack refrigerated items such as fruits, vegetables, and proteins. Check with your airline (and your country of destination if you're going abroad) for guidelines on packing a carry-on cooler.

✔ Before leaving on your trip, search for health food stores located near where you're staying. You may find that healthy, wheat-free options are just around the corner if you're in a pinch.

When traveling internationally, be it business or leisure, additional challenges arise. The most glaring one may be a language barrier. Confusion often results when you're trying to convey your desire for a wheat-free meal to someone who doesn't speak your language. Finding restaurant employees who can understand you is vital in these circumstances. If possible, seek out these restaurants before you leave on your trip.

Preparing your own meals even when traveling

Your destination, your accommodations, and the purpose of your travels determine how feasibly you can prepare your own meals. When renting a house on the beach, a condo near the ski slopes, or cabin in the woods, a trip to the local health food grocery store is all you need to prepare the wheat-free meal you desire. When visiting friends, offer to help in the kitchen by cooking one or more meals. Your host will love you for earning your keep.

Unfortunately, if your travels involve accommodations that don't have a place to prepare meals, you may be out of luck. You may find gluten-free pre-made meals at the local health food grocery store. And prepared snacks can act as a meal in emergency situations (though that's not the best-case scenario).

Chapter 15

Navigating Special Occasions

In This Chapter

▶ Preparing for family gatherings and holiday celebrations

▶ Keeping tabs on your food choices at work functions

▶ Interacting with others about your wheat-free diet

Some of the most challenging times you experience on your wheat-free journey include eating with people who haven't seen the wheat-free light (at least not yet). What do you do when meal preparation is completely out of your hands or traditional holiday foods that don't fit your lifestyle surround you at every turn?

Now isn't the time to be shy about your pledge to a wheat-free lifestyle. You don't have to flaunt your new health commitment, but you should be prepared for whatever dining experience you may encounter. Let others know that you've gone wheat-free and that it will impact the foods you eat. Doing so will cut down on the amount of stress you feel when you turn down food that is offered to you.

Assuming you've gone wheat-free by personal preference (not on doctor's orders because of a health condition such as celiac disease), not all is necessarily lost if you give in and live it up a little during a wheat-filled holiday or social gathering. The pressures to succumb, the inconvenience of finding food alternatives when they're not immediately available, and the desire not to burden other people attending your gathering are all legitimate reasons for easing off your wheat-free diet for a meal. Just don't use that as an excuse for an extended break.

In this chapter, we explain a couple of schools of thought regarding wheat-free strictness and offer tips on how to enjoy celebrations without completely blowing your diet. We discuss some proactive measures and modifications you can make to ensure you eat what you want to. You also find guidance on how to plan a successful wheat-free experience when you're dining with others who aren't wheat-free, including your boss and other colleagues, and the healthiest food seems miles away. Finally, we help you respond to tough wheat-free questions and comments that are destined to come your way from friends, family members, and coworkers.

Attending Family Celebrations and Holiday Events

Celebrations and holidays have a way of dragging on for days and weeks, and they can wreak havoc on your diet if you're not ready. Think about all the wedding showers, parties, and dinners leading up to the big event, or that whole gauntlet from Thanksgiving through Hanukkah, Christmas, and New Year's. With all the biscuits, breads, stuffings, gravies, cakes, pies — you name it — it's a wonder anyone resurfaces after the celebration unscathed. But if you create a plan and stick to it, you'll survive the feeding frenzy.

If you slip up, make sure you know your wheat consumption limits. Over-indulging can have serious consequences based on your level of wheat sensitivity. If you have a tolerable reaction to wheat and accidentally eat too much, allow yourself a break and give yourself permission to cheat a little bit knowing that, as soon as the celebration is over, you'll return to your wheat-free diet. This flexibility can alleviate feelings of deprivation as long as you manage it realistically.

One of the worst things you can do is beat yourself up over a wheat indiscretion. This negativity can lead to frustration and even to your quitting your wheat-free lifestyle altogether. Even the strongest people make mistakes; just own it and get back on track quickly. Don't let your celebrations linger from a dietary standpoint.

Deciding between strict avoidance and the occasional indulgence

We recommend a cold-turkey approach to removing wheat (and really, all grains) from your diet because of the addictive and comforting effect they have; if you let them linger as you phase them out, you may have trouble getting rid of them completely. After they're gone, though, you may be able to handle letting a little back in on occasion. Knowing your ability to bounce back after a holiday or celebratory wheat splurge is crucial in determining how far you can or can't go when you face the possibility of going off the wagon. The following sections depict how two types of people who eliminate wheat from their diet approach festivities and get-togethers. Those people are the doers and the relaxers.

The doers

Doers are people who are driven to maintain their wheat-free lifestyles. On the rare occasions that they cheat on their diets, they usually pass over the mistake and quickly forget after a short mourning spell has passed. Doers insist on taking their own lunches to work, to school, on vacation, and even to other people's homes if they're not convinced they'll have a wheat-free meal waiting for them. They're constantly planning ahead and staying on top of their diets.

Friends, family, and coworkers are usually aware of the doers' habits because wheat-free eating is one of those defining characteristics that overflow into other areas of their lives. Doers can sometimes come across as preachy and judgmental, but usually that's just a matter of their passion for spreading the wheat-free message.

As you may have guessed, doers continue to eliminate all wheat products even during holidays and family celebrations when gluten-filled food is in abundance. From food gifts and stocking stuffers to rehearsal dinners and receptions, doers remain committed to their cause. People tell the doer, "You're so strong. I don't know how you do it," and, "I wish I had your willpower," which encourages more of the same behavior.

The relaxers

Relaxers are similar to doers in that they're deeply committed to their wheat-free lifestyles. But whereas doers can seem preachy, relaxers tend to inspire those around them rather than discourage. Relaxers navigate food choices

---

Letting your body determine your limits

"How far do I have to go with my wheat-free lifestyle for it to be considered wheat-free?" and "Can't I fudge just a little bit from time to time on my wheat-free diet?" are common questions among those making the switch to wheat-free living.

These are great questions that can only be answered by your reaction to wheat and grains and what you're willing to put up with. If you're not bothered or are only slightly affected by inflammation, digestive issues, weight gain, or allergies, you may be willing to be less strict with the amount of wheat you eat.

However, eating wheat prevents you from looking and feeling your healthiest. Most people who endure low-grade levels of allergies, inflammation, weight gain, and digestive problems chalk them up to some other cause and say, "That's just a part of life," and, "I'm just getting older." They're not aware that wheat is at the root of their problems.

Warning: Of course, if you suffer from celiac disease, the answers to these questions are pretty clear: Wheat is off the menu, period. (Flip to Chapter 3 for more on celiac disease and wheat.)

in an unassuming way that isn't arrogant or rude. Simply put, they become dietary role models for those considering a change to a wheat- or grain-free program.

When family celebrations and holidays roll around, relaxers are much more flexible in their food choices than doers. They may sneak a piece of wedding cake, have a serving of stuffing and gravy, and eat a chocolate Santa or two out of their stockings, but they don't go crazy with their diets. They're more willing to make exceptions here and there to fit family celebration and holiday traditions. This approach causes little to no stress to those involved.

Finding the right balance

Are you a doer or a relaxer? If you said "some of both," then you're right on track. Doers are strong in their determination as they stay on the path. They attend weddings, reunions, and graduations without a dietary blemish and emerge from holidays with a diet worthy of a five-star rating.

However, the doer's attitude can be dampening to others. No one likes to feel judged or preached to. This kind of interaction turns people off before they even have a chance to hear the benefits of living the wheat-free lifestyle.

Relaxers appear to have a handle on the wheat they consume. They mesh seamlessly at family celebrations and on holidays because of their flexibility. They're never an inconvenience to a host. Their nonabrasive approach is often a good recruiter to the wheat-free lifestyle.

However, a too-lax approach, especially during the holidays, can lead to a downward spiral disaster for relaxers. Having to change back to a wheat-free diet from your culinary debauchery can be quite difficult when you've gone too far off track.

We recommend a happy-medium approach between the two wheat-free dietary styles. Your personality strongly influences the direction you're likely to go, but becoming aware of how your lifestyle may be affecting those around you may give reason to tweak your behaviors a bit.

Eating healthfully at family and holiday celebrations

Family celebrations and holidays are a time to come together with family and friends and rejoice in the occasion. However, with these celebrations come dietary challenges that can wreak havoc on your health if you don't confront them. An awareness of these challenges and how they affect you is the first step in heading them off at the pass:

- ✔ **Copious amounts of easily accessible food:** From the proverbial fruit-cake in the mail to wedding cake and tables of buffet food, food is often a central part of celebratory occasions.

- ✔ **Emotional eating:** Most people eat in response to their emotional states. Indulging a bit at a family gathering to be part of the festivities is one thing; retreating to the snack table to nurse your hurt feelings when an old family conflict reignites is another.

- ✔ **Excuses/coping mechanisms:** Statements like "I'm too busy right now. I'll get back to my diet and exercise program after the holidays," and "It's the holidays; let's just celebrate!" are ways of allowing yourself to splurge. Relying on them too heavily for justification can spell major trouble if you don't have the discipline to bounce back quickly from an indulgence.

- ✔ **Fear of social confrontation:** "Try one of my cupcakes," or "I don't want to eat this by myself!" is a subtle way for a friend or family member to put pressure on you. This type of pressure can overwhelm the best of intentions. In some cultures, refusing food that's offered is specifically considered impolite or rude, a situation that can compound this fear even more.

- ✔ **Stress:** The body produces the hormone *cortisol* in response to elevated stress levels, and cortisol stimulates a desire for sweets. Celebrations and family time can be major stressors (financially, emotionally, and logistically), so be aware of how this stress may influence your food choices.

- ✔ **Lack of sleep:** Insufficient sleep increases insulin resistance and the production of cortisol, which contribute to your food choices and your level of hunger.

- ✔ **Different standards for special days and the everyday:** Most people view special occasions differently from their daily grinds. This discrepancy is often what they use to justify having separate sets of guidelines when it comes to food choices.

Most people experience some or all of these issues when dealing with family celebrations and holidays. Thankfully, relief is in sight. Here are some ideas to help you devise a wheat-free plan that will help you emerge victorious when it's all over:

- ✔ **Plan ahead.** Eating at home before or after the celebration gives you total control over what you eat. By eating before the event, you lessen the temptation to overindulge in wheat-filled offerings. If you plan on eating a full meal at home after the celebration, you may want to have a snack before the party to make sure you don't get too hungry.

✔ **Bring a dish.** If you'll be a guest at someone else's celebration, offer to bring one or two of your favorite wheat-free dishes. This approach ensures you'll have some wheat-free options.

✔ **Drink plenty of water.** Make sure you're adequately hydrated leading up to the big celebration (and throughout the holiday season in general). People often mistake thirst for hunger; drinking a glass of water can often put the kibosh on wheat cravings.

✔ **Create new, healthier family food traditions.** Find wheat-free recipes that resemble traditional holiday and party foods and add them to your spread. Pretty soon, the old wheat standbys will be a distant memory. For example, the Prosciutto-Wrapped Asparagus and Goat Cheese (Chapter 11), Jalapeños in a Bacon Blanket (Chapter 12), and Cashew Butter and Chocolate Chip Cookies (Chapter 13) are wonderful substitutes for your usual holiday fare.

✔ **Eat the healthiest wheat-free options first.** Whenever you're a guest at someone else's gathering, eat the wheat-free foods first. You may find they're enough to satisfy your hunger.

✔ **Practice mindful eating.** With each bite, focus on how the food looks, smells, tastes, and feels (its texture). By taking the time to focus on each bite, you're less likely to eat something that you weren't planning to.

✔ **Leave the table when you're done.** When possible, remove yourself from the table after you finish eating the healthiest food at the celebration so you won't be tempted to eat the next course, which is usually wheat-filled desserts. If leaving the table isolates you from the rest of the group, offer to help clear off the table of dishes and food as everyone's eating dessert. Doing so removes you from the social obligation of eating dessert without making you seem standoffish.

✔ **Recognize and avoid emotional eating.** Holidays and special occasions have a way of stirring up both positive and negative emotions. Pay close attention to how your eating patterns are affected by these emotions.

✔ **Host your own gathering.** Even though planning an event sounds stressful, it gives you total control over what will be served at your house. Designing a wheat/grain-free menu not only eliminates your snacking on off-limits foods during preparation but also increases your options during the celebration.

If your guests insist on contributing dishes that may contain wheat, politely insist that they take their leftovers with them when they leave.

✔ **Watch your alcohol consumption.** Drinking too much may impair your decision making process, leading you to eat foods that you may not ordinarily eat. (Plus, some alcohols contain gluten, which is problematic if you've eliminated wheat because of a gluten sensitivity or intolerance.)

Tackling Work Functions and Business Dinners

Work functions and business dinners are for gathering with coworkers you seldom see, landing the next big deal, developing your business knowledge base, and impressing the boss. The last thing you need to be stressed out about is what you're going to eat. Although some company meal planners consider every possible food recommendation from attendees, you can't afford to take this accommodation for granted. You must be proactive in your approach to your next business dinner.

Whether you're planning events or attend them, the issue of food preparation is extremely important to your and other attendees' health. In the next sections, we give you some pointers for planning meals and events that take into account people's special dietary needs and help you navigate gatherings planned by others.

Accommodating wheat-free needs when hosting a business meal or event

When choosing a restaurant or planning the menu for a meeting, sales pitch, or event that includes food, you must consider the other attendees' dietary requirements. Your consideration allows the attendees an opportunity to enjoy the meal and eliminates the temptations to straying from their wheat-free diet.

In the planning stage, ask those who will be attending whether they have any food requirements. Have attendees fill out a food questionnaire, and then follow up with them by phone to make sure you're clear on their dietary needs. Do everything you can to accommodate those requests. If you're not sure whether the foods you've selected will suit your guests' needs, ask the restaurant or caterer for guidance on which foods are wheat-free. (Chapter 14 shows you what questions to ask to determine whether an establishment can meet wheat-free needs.)

Receptions can be one of the more challenging occasions to plan. Heavy hors d'oeuvres are a popular reception food that doesn't exactly give you a whole bunch of options. As the host, though, always work to provide at least one wheat-free option for your guests. Your wheat-free guests will appreciate it.

If you're throwing a birthday or retirement party or a wedding or baby shower for one of your coworkers, be considerate of the fact that others in attendance may be wheat- or gluten-free. Provide a wheat-free treat for those who may prefer that option. Some wheat-free party foods are so delicious that your party attendees may not even know they're guiltlessly indulging. (Check out Part III for some tasty wheat-free options.)

Attending a business meal or event where food will be served

When you're invited to a breakfast or lunch meeting, business dinner, or other business event involving food, you have some options for sticking to your wheat-free diet:

- ✔ **Let the organizer know that you need a wheat-free meal.** If your request isn't well received, offer to help with the meal planning. If your assistance is refused, don't give up. Try one of the following options.

- ✔ **Eat before the meeting or event.** A wheat-free snack such as a hard-boiled egg and fruit may be enough to tide you over until you can eat a full meal after your meeting. When people ask why you're not eating, explain that you already ate.

- ✔ **Eat after the meeting or event.** When people ask why you're not eating, say that you're not hungry if you don't want to discuss your choice to live wheat-free. (If the meeting may be a long one, consider having a snack beforehand.)

- ✔ **Call ahead to see whether the restaurant can accommodate your food preferences.** If you can order your own meal for the meeting, you're home-free.

Satisfying your stomach at conferences

When attending large sales meetings or conferences, look for questions about dietary requirements on the registration form. They're your opportunity to express your wheat- or grain-free needs. If the registration form doesn't ask about the need for special meals, make sure you convey that information to the event coordinator some other way.

Most coordinators carefully plan out the menu to feed the masses and address each special dietary requirement individually. If you don't make your needs known, chances are you won't have wheat-free meals waiting for you at the conference. When conferences are held at facilities that don't have kitchens, it's very difficult for the caterer to accommodate someone who hasn't pre-ordered a wheat-free meal.

Often times, conference coordinators hand you a colored card at check-in that indicates you stated a wheat-free food preference. Placing this card at your table ensures a wheat-free meal will be delivered to you when you're seated.

Sometimes you attend a meeting or conference where the meal is served buffet style. More than likely, you'll find wheat- or grain-free options, but be extremely careful of cross-contamination. Facilities don't always pay close attention to transferring food from place to place, and serving utensils in the various dishes are sure to get moved from dish to dish without regard for wheat content.

Celebrating milestones with coworkers

If you attend a celebratory event like a birthday party or baby shower and no wheat-free choices are available, you have a few options that don't have to draw attention to your situation:

- ✔ Skip out on the cake or cookies with the explanation that you're on a wheat-free diet and trying to stay strong in your commitment to it. If you know that the temptation will be great, bring a prepared wheat-free treat for yourself.

- ✔ Politely take some of the treats to your desk and privately dispose of them without eating any.

- ✔ If you find out about the party at the last second, walk into the room eating a healthy, wheat-free snack. You'll get a pass when you finish your snack and say you're full.

Although some people may be out to sabotage your dietary efforts, stay the course. Many people will try to persuade you by saying, "Here, have a small piece," or "Bernice made this; it's to die for!" Whatever the temptation, exercise self-control.

Managing the open bar

Whether you're meeting for drinks after work or over a business dinner to close a deal, alcohol is usually at the center of the gathering. Calling the bar or restaurant to see whether it's equipped to meet your wheat-free needs and/or you can bring your own bottle lets you stay wheat-free and enjoy a glass of your favorite alcoholic beverage.

The temptation to drink at these functions can be very strong. If you're not prepared, you may find yourself in trouble, especially if you're highly sensitive to wheat or gluten. Even though avoiding wheat when having a drink is possible, remember that many mixed drinks contain sugary juices that greatly affect your blood sugar and insulin levels.

When you want to enjoy an adult beverage, here's what to be on the lookout for in each of the three categories of alcohol:

- ✔ **Beer:** Beer is wheat-free but not gluten-free, so if you're not avoiding gluten, beer is an okay option. Traditionally, beer is made with barley, which contains gluten. However, brewers are now using buckwheat, millet, and sorghum in place of barley to remove the gluten. Gluten-free beers can be difficult to find because of their seasonal and regional limitations. If a restaurant doesn't carry what you're looking for, you may want to consider one of its gluten-free alcoholic options. (For details on how wheat-free is different from gluten-free, check out Chapter 3.)

- ✔ **Liquor:** Presumably, distillation eliminates gluten from the wheat, barley, and rye that's used in making gin, vodka, and whiskey, creating a gluten-free drink. However, some makers don't fully distill the alcohol to the point that all the gluten is removed, and some add gluten-containing grain to give the drink a more palatable flavor and color.

    Although most hard liquor is considered safe, if you suffer from celiac disease or are gluten intolerant, you may want to err on the side of caution. Look for non-grain liquors such as brandy, rum, tequila, potato-based vodka, and juniper berry-based gin.

- ✔ **Wine:** Wine is made from the fermentation of grapes and therefore is generally regarded as being wheat- and gluten-free. However, some wine makers add food coloring and flavoring that contains wheat, age their wine in barrels that contain wheat paste, or use wheat to fine their wine for clarity and sediment removal. Added colors and flavors are usually found in dessert wines that have a strong fruit flavor. If you look hard enough, you can find organic wines that are free of these practices and additives, rendering them wheat-free.

Most restaurants won't give you an ingredient list for drinks unless you ask. Even then, they may be reluctant to give out any recipe secrets. When in doubt, play it safe and stick to beverages you know to be wheat-free.

Talking about Your Dietary Choices with Others

Having conversations about your new wheat-free diet can become one of the most rewarding and frustrating aspects of your change experience. Some people will ask you legitimate scientific questions, while others will ask condescending questions and mock your answers.

The types of questions we typically get refer to the effects wheat has on our health. The trick is to answer them in layperson's terms as much as possible; if we get too scientific about blood sugar and insulin, inflammation, and so on, the listener starts to glaze over.

Basically, the argument is for eating unprocessed *whole foods* such as meats, fish, chicken, eggs, fruits, and vegetables. The greatest challenge is using this information. The "healthy whole-grain" diet idea is driven by conventional wisdom, so debunking this way of thinking can take multiple conversations. But as people listen to your logic and see the positive changes brought on by your daily wheat-free diet, they're more likely to listen to you and experiment with it. Your personal example of a wheat-free lifestyle is the strongest testimony you can give

It never pays to be pushy. Knowledge is power; the more you know, the more easily you can correct inaccurate beliefs. But overloading people with information or giving the appearance of force-feeding them the anti-wheat ideal will only turn them off. Be gentle in your answers.

It can also be quite irritating when people mock your efforts to educate them or give you a blank stare when the wheat topic comes up. You never really know what they're thinking. If you're being ridiculed for your dietary choices, there comes a point when the conversation is no longer productive. At this point, change the subject. The last thing you want is for a friend or family member to avoid you because they're tired of your message.

In the following sections, we present common questions and statements you're likely to hear when someone finds out you live a wheat-free lifestyle. We follow each one with information you can use to satisfy other people's curiosity.

"Where do you get your fiber, vitamins, and minerals?"

As we explain in Chapter 4, you actually get significantly more fiber, vitamins, and minerals from fruits and vegetables than from wheat. Insoluble fiber's only real purpose is to spread out the benefits of the fermentable soluble fiber and move along the digestion process. Of course, this "advantage" comes with wheat's harmful effects. Whole wheat's vitamin and mineral content is a bit misleading anyway; several minerals such as calcium, iron, zinc, and magnesium are blocked from absorption. This malabsorption can lead to nutrient deficiencies and a whole list of other problems.

Some foods you can substitute for wheat as fiber and nutrient sources are almonds, avocados, beans, broccoli, lentils, prunes, spinach, and squash. All these whole foods are rich in fiber, vitamins, and minerals and are quickly absorbed by the body. You can buy these and other healthy wheat alternatives in the organic section at your local grocery or health food store.

"What about healthy whole grains in the USDA food pyramid?"

The USDA Food Guide Pyramid, which was drawn up in 1992, suggested that Americans eat 6 to 11 servings per day from the grain group. The pyramid setup has since been abandoned in favor of the MyPlate model unveiled in 2011. However, one-quarter of the plate is still set aside for grains, breads, cereals, and pasta.

MyPlate still places the focus on eating grains, which lead to many of the chronic illnesses we see today. In a perfect world, grains would disappear from the MyPlate recommendations much like sugar has. Healthy fats would have a significant presence — at least 50 percent of the calories consumed — with protein, fruits, vegetables, and dairy filling out the rest of the plate. The fruit section would be much smaller than the current model.

"You must have a problem with wheat. I don't."

Most experts agree that wheat gluten affects everyone; it just depends to what degree. For some people, the slightest amount of wheat can lead to an extremely dangerous situation; others simply experience a low-grade allergy that they blame on something in the air. Most people probably fall somewhere between those two extremes.

Many people don't realize they have a problem with wheat because they've never seen how their bodies behave without it. This unawareness is common in several areas of health where consequences don't immediately follow poor health choices. Take the example of someone who doesn't believe he has a vision problem until he gets glasses and realizes how much better he can see.

When symptoms occur after weeks, months, or even years of a particular behavior, it's very easy to blame the symptoms on some other cause. This tendency makes identifying the problem very difficult. I, Rusty, often suggest my clients remove wheat and grains from their diets for a period of time to see what changes they notice. Usually, the changes are significant and include weight loss, more energy, fewer allergies, less joint pain, and fewer or no gastric and digestive problems.

"I think everything in moderation."

When people play the "everything in moderation" card, what they're really saying is, "I can't give up wheat." or "I'd rather not debate you on the problems associated with eating wheat." They're trying to end the conversation as politely as they can because they feel they're comfortable with their current lifestyle. Your best bet is to simply change the subject and make your wheat-free case by letting your actions and improved health speak for you.

"Moderation" is often an attempt to rationalize behavior by flirting with disaster. After all, when was the last time you had only one potato chip or cookie? The term *moderation* itself is relative anyway. What one person considers moderate may seem excessive to another and minimal to a third.

"All of my favorite foods are loaded with wheat. I couldn't give them up."

This comment is a cousin to the standby "Eating wheat-free/grain-free is too restrictive." At first, most people struggle with the idea of giving up delicious wheat-filled treats. To some, it's an insurmountable task because of wheat's addictive qualities. The reason they believe they can't stop eating those foods is because they continue to eat them. The more they eat them, the more they want them.

In reality, eating wheat-free is liberating. When you eliminate wheat from your diet, you don't crave it anymore. That may sound crazy at first, but you develop a taste for other healthy, wheat-free foods. Plenty of tasty and healthy wheat-free foods are out there that you've probably never experienced. You also notice an increase in energy, a loss of bloating and gastric distress, a feeling of satiation, and possible weight loss.

"I've been wheat-free for a while, and I haven't lost any weight to speak of."

When you eat naturally wheat-free food, you diminish the fat storing effects of elevated blood sugar. By decreasing your carbohydrate intake, you keep your insulin production low, and your body burns fat as your primary fuel source. This shift usually leads to weight loss. However, the degree to which you metabolize carbohydrates directly affects how much weight you lose.

If you're not losing the amount of weight you want, a couple of possibilities exist:

- ✔ **You may be eating foods with hidden wheat and sugar.** Everybody metabolizes carbohydrates differently, such that some can lose weight by just reducing their carbohydrate intake, whereas others must eliminate carbs altogether to see the changes they're looking for. (For help identifying sneaky names for wheat and sugar, flip to Chapter 7.)

  To combat this problem, start by eliminating all the carbohydrates in your diet. After you're carb-free and have lost some weight, slowly add individual carbohydrates back into your diet to see which and how many carbohydrates you can tolerate.

- ✔ **In your effort to cut wheat and sugar, you may have upped your protein intake rather than your fat intake.** For many, the word *fat* still leads to images of clogged arteries, so they shy away from it and load up on protein instead. But too much protein leads to glucose production, which creates a similar blood sugar response to that of a high-wheat/ high-sugar diet.

  If you have this problem, the solution may be starting a high-fat diet. When you consume about 70 to 80 percent of your calories from healthy fats, your body begins to accumulate ketones in your bloodstream. *Ketones* are a byproduct of fat metabolism; your body becomes a fat-burning machine by using these ketones (not glucose) for fuel. The remaining 20 to 30 percent of your calories come from protein and carbohydrates.

If you try these approaches and you still don't see the scale change, fear not; it doesn't mean that your efforts are for naught. Weight loss isn't the only advantage to living wheat-free. The "unseen" benefits are well documented. Your inflammation levels improve, you reduce your joint pain and allergies, and much, much more. Most of these benefits are difficult to specifically identify without a blood test, elimination diet, or allergy test, but using these markers will only confirm your improved feeling of well-being.

Chapter 16

A Workout That Works

*O*ne of the toughest things to do is carve out time in your already-hectic schedule to exercise. But it's one of the most important. Consider the following:

✔ According to the American Diabetes Association, 25.6 million people have diabetes, and 79 million people have pre-diabetes (2011 National Diabetes Fact Sheet).

✔ According to the Heart Foundation, about 1 million people die annually of heart disease. By 2020, it'll be the leading cause of death worldwide.

✔ According to Cancer.org, 33 percent of all women and 50 percent of all men will develop cancer.

✔ According to the Centers for Disease Control and Prevention, 3.4 percent of Americans suffer from deep depression, and 9 percent experience an occasional bout of depression.

No, exercise isn't the cure-all for everything listed, but a regular exercise program can reduce the likelihood that you'll fall into one of those categories, and it will also improve how you feel and boost your confidence. Who doesn't want that?

Like it or not, your health is directly related to the lifestyle choices you make on a daily basis. What you eat, how much sleep you get, and how you manage stress are all very important to a healthy life. But have you ever considered how exercise fits into living a wheat/grain-free life?

In this chapter, we explain the benefits of doing various types of exercise while living wheat-free. We discuss what you need to consider when determining what you want to achieve with your exercise program. Then we offer some specific exercises that you can incorporate into a resistance training program that fits your individual needs.

Understanding How Exercise Enriches a Wheat-Free Lifestyle

Two areas of your wellness, glucose tolerance/insulin resistance and stress reduction, are directly related to wheat consumption and exercise. Here's how it works: When you eat wheat, the carbohydrates in the wheat are converted to glucose and stored in the liver, muscles, and fat tissue. When multiple glucose molecules bind together, they're called *glycogen*. The rest of the glucose floats around in your bloodstream waiting for the hormone insulin to escort it to a muscle or fat cell to be used as energy at a later time. (The pancreas secretes insulin in response to the carbohydrates you consume.)

You become insulin resistant (glucose intolerant) when you have too much insulin in the bloodstream and your cells no longer welcome the glucose. At that point, excessive blood sugar and insulin levels can create many chronic illnesses, including obesity, Type 2 diabetes, heart disease, many cancers, gout, and Alzheimer's disease.

Regular, vigorous exercise several times a week improves glucose tolerance and can reduce insulin resistance by increasing insulin sensitivity. Actually, it can prevent and reverse the effects of insulin resistance before you reach one of the related diseases.

Exercise also helps lower the effects of stress on your health. Your body was built to handle stress in order to get you out of dangerous situations. However, it wasn't designed to handle one stressful episode after another without a break. This continuous state of stress leads to elevated cortisol levels (*cortisol* is the primary stress hormone secreted by your body). In turn, high cortisol levels contribute to a multitude of potential health problems, including anxiety, heart disease, hyperglycemia (high blood sugar), high blood pressure, sleep problems, and weight gain.

When they're under ongoing stress, many people reach for comfort food to help ease the stress and calm the nerves. From soups to pizza, these foods are typically laden with wheat- or grain-filled ingredients. You can see where this is going.

A healthier way to deal with stress is to exercise. Exercise increases cortisol levels for the duration of each workout, but regular moderate-to-intense exercise lowers cortisol levels overall. Also, the more you exercise, the less you'll want to eat unhealthy, wheat-filled foods for fear of undoing all your hard work in the gym. If you must eat during a stressful situation, choose a healthy, wheat- or grain-free food; otherwise, you're just adding insult to injury.

If these reasons aren't enough to get you to throw on your sweats and get moving, here are a few more exercise benefits to think about:

✔ Improves brain function and cardiovascular/cardio-respiratory fitness

✔ Improves energy levels, mood, and sleep

✔ Prevents osteoporosis

✔ Reduces stress and anxiety

✔ Strengthens muscles, bones, and joints

Getting Started on a New, Fit You

Don't let the title of this section fool you. You don't need a New Year's resolution to get started on the "new you." All you need is a desire to change and a willingness to learn. Many times, a change in lifestyle behavior is brought on by a health scare or the realization that life is more enjoyable when you follow healthy lifestyle behaviors. Regardless of your impetus to change, act on it as soon as possible.

Consult with your physician before starting any kind of exercise program. Your doctor will be able to identify whether you have any areas of health you should be cautious with.

Determining your needs

If living a happy, healthy, and fit life is on your to-do list, determining your needs isn't so difficult. Everyone can stand to benefit from a well-designed workout and dietary program. The question is, how do you know what you need? Well, consider some of the following health markers and risk numbers:

✔ Blood pressure higher than 140/90 mm/Hd

✔ Body mass index (BMI) of 30 or higher

✔ Fasting blood glucose levels higher than 100 mg/dL

✔ HDL (good) cholesterol levels lower than 40 mg/dL for men and lower than 50 mg/dL for women

✔ LDL (bad) cholesterol particle numbers higher than 1,000 nmol/L (moderate risk) or higher than 2,000 nmol/L (very high risk)

✔ Triglyceride levels higher than 150 mg/dL

✔ Waist measurement of 40 inches or more for men and 35 inches or more for women

You may have other needs that have previously discouraged you from starting an exercise program. This list may include

- Joint pain caused by ligament damage
- Lack of energy
- Neck and back pain caused by poor posture
- Poor body mechanics (caused by muscle tightness) that create undue stress on various body parts

To help you identify areas that need to be attended to, ask your doctor for a physical exam and blood work-up and have a postural assessment done by a physical therapist, chiropractor, or highly trained personal trainer.

Establishing a plan of action

When you've determined what needs your fitness plan will address (see the preceding section), you're ready to plan how it will work into your schedule. Remember that working out at home will probably take less time than going to a gym, so consider travel time if necessary. Write it into your daily, weekly, and monthly calendars so you own it and it becomes part of your routine — an appointment that's not to be cancelled. People who try to wing it without a planned schedule are more likely to find reasons to put off exercising. Ask yourself these questions to decide the timing that works best for your new workout program:

- When do I have the most time during the day — before work, during my lunch hour, or after work?
- When do I tend to have the most energy — early in the morning, midday, or at the end of the day?
- What times of the day is my trainer available?
- What are the busiest times of the day at the gym?
- What days work best for me? Am I willing/available to work out on weekends?

Knowing the answers to these questions is crucial to the success of your workout program because it helps you nip the most common excuse — lack of time — in the bud.

We recommend journaling your diet and workout program. Research indicates that tracking your workout progress leads to greater awareness of and adherence to your program. It also provides tangible evidence that all your hard work is paying off. This visible sign of success feels good, increases your self-confidence, and motivates you to stick to your plan.

Write a wellness vision and set SMART goals that relate to your fitness plan. (Chapter 5 has info on establishing health visions and SMART goals.) Allowing someone else to hold you accountable is another great tool to help you avoid making excuses.

Exploring Resistance Exercises

If you're planning on working out at home, having a few yoga and Pilates videos available is a great way to get started. Or skim the exercises in the following section and pick out the ones that look most appealing to you. After you've selected the ones you want to incorporate into your routine, check out the later section "Designing Your Individualized Exercise Program" to get started.

 Start thinking of yourself as a resistance trainer, yoga or Pilates student, swimmer, cyclist, runner, or whatever. By naming yourself, you're owning the title and assuming a label you won't hesitate to refer to yourself with later. You also begin the accountability process: This label serves as an additional motivator on those

Don't sweat these myths about resistance training

The health and fitness industry is loaded with myths. Here are the most common misconceptions we hear from our clients regarding resistance training:

✔ **"I'll get bulky if I lift weights."** Typically, a normal resistance training program will strengthen your muscles but isn't going to increase their size significantly. People who develop significant amounts of muscle through resistance training usually spend much more time in the gym than what's needed for health benefits. Hormones (that is, testosterone) also play a huge factor in determining how big a person's muscles become. (That explains why men are generally bigger than women and experience greater muscle strength and size gains.) And in some cases, huge muscles are the result of performance enhancing drugs.

✔ **"I'm too busy to take the time to work out!"** The idea that you need to exercise for at least an hour every day to see results is

incorrect. Although 60 minutes is optimum, don't discount the benefits of a shorter, intense workout if that's all your schedule will allow. You can do resistance exercises at home with limited equipment or at a gym in a short period of time. Movement of any kind is always better than nothing.

✔ **"If I stop lifting, all my muscle will turn to fat!"** Muscle and fat are chemically different; one can't turn into the other. However, whatever muscle size you do gain through resistance training will be lost over time if you don't keep up the training.

✔ **"I want to exercise my stomach muscles because that's where I carry most of my fat."** This concept is known as *spot reduction,* and it doesn't work. When you exercise a muscle, you do just that — you strengthen that muscle. You don't exercise the fat between the muscle and the skin. That issue is addressed through your diet by eliminating wheat and added sugar.

days when you'd rather be doing something else. After a few weeks, you'll be in a set routine; you'll see and feel changes that will continue to motivate you.

Getting lean with weight lifting

Not only is weight lifting good exercise for your body, but it also increases your metabolism and improves your insulin sensitivity. By adding muscle mass to your body, you increase the number of calories you burn and the rate at which you burn them. Although small in number, this increase in calories burned helps keep your motor revving at a high level even at rest. Weight lifting also improves your cells' ability and availability to receive the sugar that your insulin is bringing to them to store. This helps prevent insulin resistance and the associated diseases, such as Type 2 diabetes, cancer, and heart disease.

Dumbbell Flat Press

You can perform the Dumbbell Flat Press on a flat angle or, if your exercise bench is adjustable, on an inclined angle. Both versions are a pushing movement with your chest, shoulders, and triceps as the primary movers. The inclined angle gives a bit more emphasis on the upper chest and front of the shoulders. Both angles also require the back muscles to contract to help stabilize your body throughout the movement. The form for each is the same.

1. **Sit on the bench with the dumbbells resting on your thighs, palms facing each other, as shown in Figure 16-1a.**

   Lock your elbows in their current position and lean back on the bench, taking the dumbbells with you to your shoulders.

2. **Exhale as you straighten your arms to the ceiling with your palms facing your feet.**

   Make sure your butt and upper back are pressed into the bench. Your shoulder blades are squeezed together and there should be a slight gap between your lower back and the bench. Try not to press the back of your head into the bench. See Figure 16-1b.

3. **Inhale as you lower the dumbbells to your outer chest/armpit area, creating a 90-degree angle as illustrated in Figure 16-1c.**

   Make sure your elbows are always underneath the weights for support.

4. **Press the dumbbells upward as you exhale so they come together at the top of the movement just shy of touching.**

5. **Repeat Steps 2 through 4.**

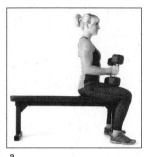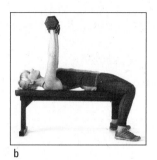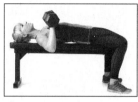

Figure 16-1:
The Dumbbell Flat Press works your chest, shoulders, and triceps.

a   b   c

Photographs by Bob McNamara

To sit back up, don't drop the dumbbells at your side; you'll strain your shoulders. Instead, after your last rep, turn your hands so your palms are facing each other. Lower the dumbbells and rest them on your chest. Lift your legs off the floor with knees bent. While rocking your legs back to the floor, tighten your abdominal muscles and crunch forward, tilting the dumbbells in the process so momentum accomplishes most of the work.

For many, getting up is the most difficult part of the exercise, so make sure you practice the proper technique with lighter weights.

One-Arm Dumbbell Row

Every group of muscles has an opposing muscle group. Whereas the Dumbbell Flat Press works the pushing muscles, the One-Arm Dumbbell Row strengthens the pulling muscles. If you've ever tried to start an old lawnmower, you know what the back muscles are good for. Lawnmower beware: The dumbbell row will make this chore and any other lifting movements quite easy.

1. **Place a dumbbell on the right side of the workout bench and position yourself so your left hand and left knee are on the bench.**

   Your right knee should be to the side, a little back and slightly bent. Stick your butt out and flatten your back while tightening your abdominal muscles. Leave a slight arch in your back so it's about parallel to the floor. Lower your chin toward your chest so you're looking at your left hand and your neck is in line with your spine.

2. **Reach down and grab the dumbbell with a loose grip as shown in Figure 16-2a.**

3. **Pull your arm up until your elbow is pointing to the ceiling as shown in Figure 16-2b.**

   Your upper arm is parallel to the ground, and your hand is between your ribcage and hip. Your forearm should be at a 90 degree angle to the floor. Keep your back flat and your abdominals contracted throughout the movement. Initiate the movement from your back, not your hand; your back is doing the moving, and your arm is just like a hook. This technique involves lifting the shoulder a bit before you even begin to move the dumbbell.

4. **Lower the weight slowly.**

5. **Repeat on the other side of the bench with your left arm.**

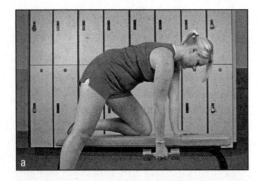

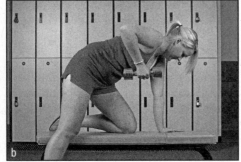

Figure 16-2: The One-Arm Dumbbell Row strengthens the back muscles.

Photographs by Matt Bowen

Push-ups

Push-ups are easy in the sense that you can do them anywhere, with no equipment necessary. They're hard in the sense that they require full body strength to accomplish the movement. Your chest, shoulders, and triceps are the primary movers, but your back and core have to step up to stabilize your planklike body position.

1. **Get on your hands and knees with your hands positioned a little wider than your shoulders and directly in line with your chest.**

2. **Lift your knees off the ground and position your body so you form a straight line from your neck to your feet, as demonstrated in Figure 16-3a.**

Don't let your back sag, but also don't stick your butt high in the air. This position is best accomplished by putting your feet about shoulder width apart and contracting your abdominal muscles. At this point, the weight of your body is being supported by your hands and the balls of your feet.

3. **Inhale while bending at the elbow and lowering your body until your elbows are at a 90-degree angle as shown in Figure 16-3b.**

   Throughout the movement, your elbows should be slightly angled back toward your feet.

4. **Exhale and straighten your elbows and return to the starting position.**

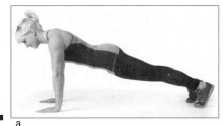

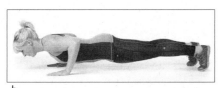

Figure 16-3:
Push-ups work your upper body, back, and core.

a

b

Photographs by Bob McNamara

If you find the movement to be painful on your wrists or elbows, consider purchasing push-up bars. These inexpensive handles should put your wrists in a better position to alleviate the pain.

If push-ups on the floor are too advanced for you, start out doing wall push-ups. Stand facing a wall with your hands slightly wider than shoulder width and follow the same directions as for floor push-ups. As the wall exercises become too easy, move to a dresser or exercise bench. Before long, you'll be on the floor doing what once seemed too difficult.

Lunges

Lunges are a fantastic exercise because they involve all the muscles of the lower body as well as a balance component. Many people are afraid lunges will hurt their knees, but done properly, lunges can become part of everyone's workout routine.

1. **Stand with your feet about shoulder width apart and take a comfortable step forward with your front foot, planting it flat on the floor and lifting your back heel off the ground.**

   Figure 16-4 shows this progression.

2. **With your chin up and eyes focused forward, bend both knees until they're almost at 90 degrees.**

   As you lower yourself, make sure your front knee remains over your ankle and doesn't extend past your toes. Extend your butt out behind you a bit to keep your front knee in proper alignment. Your back knee should be just above the ground.

Return to the starting position by pushing through the heel of your front foot. Repeat Steps 1 and 2 with one leg and then switch to the other leg.

You'll find many variations of the lunge, including walking lunges. The basic form doesn't change from lunge to lunge, so master a simple lunge and progress from there. For example, you can add dumbbells in each hand to create more resistance.

Figure 16-4:
Lunges
improve
your stability
and the
muscles in
the lower
body.

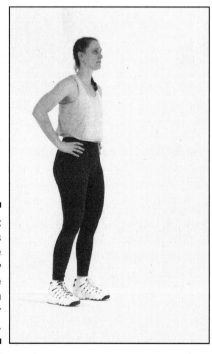 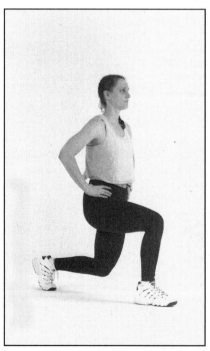

Photographs by Zoran Popovic

Squats

Like the lunge (see the preceding section), the squat is a staple for any workout routine. Squats can help improve balance and coordination as well as bone density. They also help make the simplest everyday tasks, such as getting up from a chair or bending down to pick something up, easier as you age.

1. **Stand with your feet a little wider than shoulder width apart.**

   Your arms should be at your sides; keep your chin and chest up, your shoulders back, and your eyes focused straight ahead.

2. **As you inhale, lower yourself by pushing your hips/butt backward and raise your arms out in front to counterbalance your weight. Check out Figure 16-5 for the proper form.**

   Like in the lunge, you don't want your knees to extend over your toes. If you find yourself falling backward, just lean forward a bit more. Likewise, don't let your knees bow inward while you squat. They should be in a direct line from your hips to your ankles.

   Many experts advise lowering yourself until your thighs are parallel to the ground, but we find that position to be difficult for most people and possibly stressful on the knees. Focus on lowering yourself just shy of parallel.

3. **Exhale and return to the start position by pressing with your heels and returning your arms to your sides.**

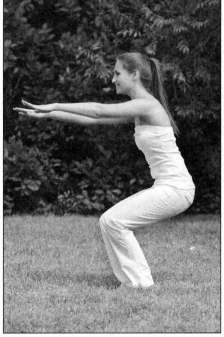

Figure 16-5:
Squats improve your balance and your bone density.

Photograph © malyugin/iStockphoto.com

Dumbbell Curls

Curls for your biceps aren't only handy for helping you lift everyday things, but they (along with tricep exercises) also make your arms more attractive in clothes.

1. **Hold a dumbbell in each hand and stand with your feet about shoulder width apart.**

   Allow your arms to hang at your sides. Stand tall, with your knees slightly bent, and tighten your abdominals by pulling them in.

2. **Lift one dumbbell until it's in front of your shoulder with your palm facing your shoulder, keeping your elbow in close to your side, as shown in Figure 16-6.**

   Don't let your elbow move forward or backward. There shouldn't be any resting at the top of the movement. Like all resistance exercises, you want constant tension on the muscle throughout.

3. **Lower the dumbbell to the starting position in a controlled manner and repeat with the other arm.**

A variation on the basic curl is called a *hammer curl*. The movement differs only in that you lift your arm straight up as if you were holding a hammer.

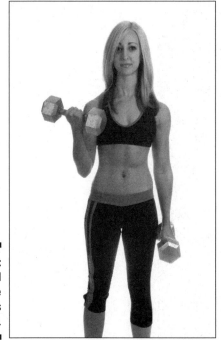

Figure 16-6:
Dumbbell
Curls make
your arms
more fit.

Photograph © RealDealPhoto/iStockphoto.com

Understanding the lever principle

Performing exercise properly is so much more than just going through the motions, even if the motions are biomechanically correct. Research has shown that when you focus on the muscle group(s) that you're working on, you generate more tension on those muscles. In other words, you get a better workout. This focus requires you to move more slowly as you perform the exercise, which cuts down on the risk of injury as well.

In order to get a deeper, more thorough understanding of how your body works while it's exercising, consider the lever principle. The *lever principle* states that the body is a system of levers separated at various points (your joints). *Tendons,* which attach muscles to bones, are the levers. When muscles contract, they create movement at the joint they cross. The lever principle states that the lever next to the lever with the resistance is doing the work. For example, the biceps muscle is the primary mover of the Dumbbell Curl exercise in this chapter because the biceps muscle crosses the elbow joint.

After you identify the primary mover of each exercise through this principle, mentally contract that muscle as you perform the exercise. As you do, you'll feel the increase in tension and stretch to that muscle throughout the range of motion of the exercise. Applying this principle to all your exercises helps you to stay mindful of and connected to your body and leads to a safer, more productive workout.

Bench Dips

The opposite muscle to the bicep is the *tricep,* which is integral in helping you lift yourself out of a chair with your arms. To work your triceps, try the Bench Dip; it requires no equipment and can be easily modified to accommodate both beginners and advanced exercisers. Additionally, your shoulders and chest benefit from this movement.

1. **Sit on the long side of a bench; place your hands on the edge of the bench right next to your hips so you're almost sitting on your thumbs.**

    Your fingertips should be able to touch the underside of the bench. Your feet should be flat on the floor in front of you with your knees bent about 90 degrees.

2. **Slide your butt off of the bench/table, as shown in Figure 16-7a, and with your abdominals pulled in, bend your elbows to lower your body toward the floor.**

    Be sure to keep your hips and back very close to the bench. Many people rub the side of the support so they don't stray too far away. Also, your elbows should be pointing backward as you move, not out to the side. Continue lowering yourself until your elbows are bent about 90 degrees, as shown in Figure 16-7b.

3. **Return to the starting position by pushing down on the bench until your arms are straight.**

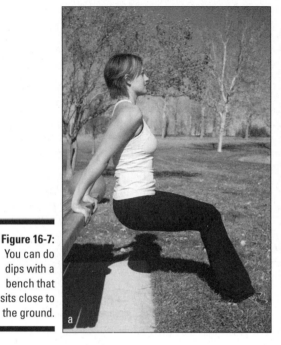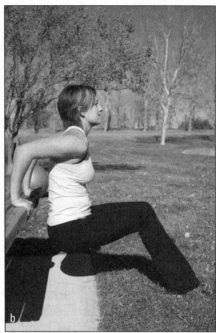

Figure 16-7: You can do dips with a bench that sits close to the ground.

Photographs © indykb/iStockphoto.com

You can easily make this exercise more difficult by relying less on help from your legs. Simply extend your feet straight in front of you with no bend in the knee. Point your toes to the ceiling so your heels are dug into the floor and perform the exercise as described earlier.

Gaining strength with core exercises

By strengthening your core muscles — those found in the abdominal, lower back, hips, pelvis, and gluteal areas — you greatly diminish your chances of developing back pain, something that affects many people at some point during their lives. Core muscles help to support and stabilize the pelvic region and promote good posture. Weak core muscles invite poor posture and an inability to protect against the stresses placed on your core, which often leads to injury.

Pilates Modified Hundred Abdominal Exercise

This exercise is a beginning Pilates movement designed to strengthen your core. The body position of this movement allows beginners to feel safe while still challenging an advanced exerciser.

1. **Lie on your back with your legs raised and knees bent about 90 degrees as Figure 16-8a illustrates.**

2. **With your arms extended at shoulder height and palms down, exhale and lift your head and shoulders off the ground (see Figure 16-8b).**

3. **Inhale as you pump your arms up and down five times, then exhale and pump your arms five more times.**

4. **Lower your head and shoulders back to the ground.**

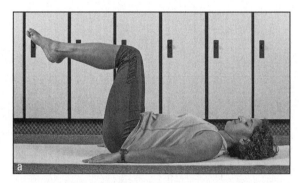

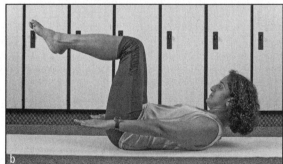

Figure 16-8:
The Pilates Modified Hundred Abdominal Exercise gives your core a good workout.

Photographs by Matt Bowen

Pilates One-Leg Teaser

This exercise, like most Pilates movements, requires strength, flexibility, and control. It's a great foundation builder for tackling more advanced Pilates moves if that interests you.

1. **Lie on your back with your feet flat on the floor and your knees bent at 90 degrees.**

2. **Extend your arms to the ceiling with your palms facing each other.**

3. **Extend your right leg so it's in line with your left thigh, pointing your toes.**

4. **Exhale as you slowly lift your head and shoulders off of the ground reaching toward your extended ankle as shown in Figure 16-9a.**

5. **Inhale then exhale as you lower yourself back to the ground as shown in Figure 16-9b.**

Figure 16-9:
The Pilates
One-Leg
Toooor
increases
your
flexibility.

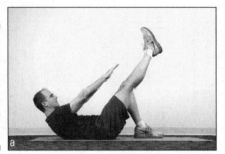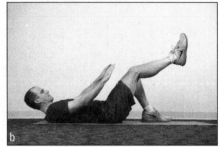

Photographs by Matt Bowen

Plank

On the surface, planks look to be a fairly simple exercise, but looks can be deceiving. When done properly, planks are extremely challenging. Mastering them is worth the effort, though, because they improve core stability. Your arms, spine, and legs benefit as well, resulting in good posture and fewer back injuries.

1. **Assume a push-up position with your elbows bent 90 degrees so you're resting on both forearms as shown in Figure 16-10.**

   Your elbows should be directly under your shoulders, with your head in a neutral position to your spine. Keeping your eyes on your hands should set up this head position naturally. You want to create a straight line from your head to your feet to fully engage the abdominal muscles. You should have the feeling of sucking in your stomach to achieve the abdominal contraction required throughout the exercise.

2. **Hold this position for the designated length of time.**

   Aim for 15 seconds at first with the ultimate goal being 90 seconds. Don't be discouraged if you can't hold the correct position for very long. Your ability to maintain this position will increase with each successive workout.

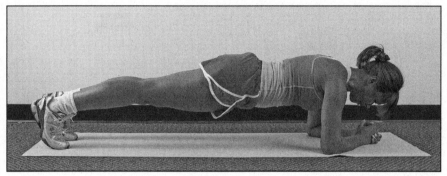

Photograph by Matt Bowen

Figure 16-10:
The Plank helps improve your posture.

Side Plank

Another staple of your exercise routine is the side plank, a variation of the regular plank in the preceding section. This version emphasizes slightly different muscles — mainly the oblique muscles.

1. **Lie on your right side with your legs straight and your left leg stacked on top of your right leg.**

   Bend your right elbow and place it directly under your shoulder. Your forearm should be perpendicular to your body.

2. **Tighten your abdominals and lift your hips off of the ground to form a direct line from your head to your feet as shown in Figure 16-11.**

   Only the side of your right foot and your forearm/elbow should be in contact with the ground. Always keep your hips square and your neck in line with your spine.

   If this position is too difficult, start by bending your knees throughout the hold, creating a straight line from your knee to your shoulder. Your lower legs should be at a 90-degree angle to your upper thighs. Your right knee should be on the ground with your left knee stacked on top. The bent-knee position is easier because you reduce the amount of tension on the obliques (the muscles that run along the sides of your rib cage).

3. **Hold for the recommended amount of time; lower yourself to the ground and repeat on your left side.**

   Beginners should start with a 15-second hold with your knees bent and work up to holding the position for 30 seconds. Once there, move to the straight-leg position for 15 seconds, working up to 30 seconds.

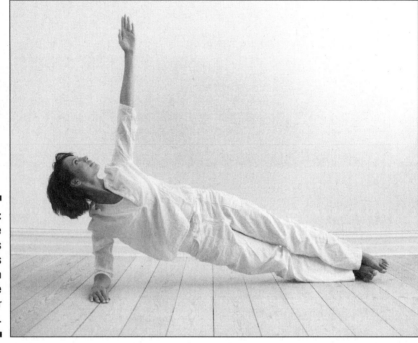

Figure 16-11:
The Side Plank tones the muscles that run along the sides of your trunk.

Back Extensions

The modern lifestyle has people sitting more — hunched in front of a computer, driving a car, lying on the sofa, and so on. This position inevitably causes posture and back issues, so Back Extensions are an important exercise to counteract these ill effects.

1. **Lie on your stomach with your arms outstretched in front of you, palms down, and your legs straight out behind you.**

2. **Lift your left arm and right leg at the same time (as demonstrated in Figure 16-12), making sure your lower back is doing the initial lifting.**

   Just an inch or two off the floor is enough.

3. **Briefly pause and lower your arm and leg to the ground.**

4. **Alternate arms and legs in a controlled manner for the desired number of repetitions.**

Figure 16-12:
Back
Extensions
strengthen
the muscles
around the
spine.

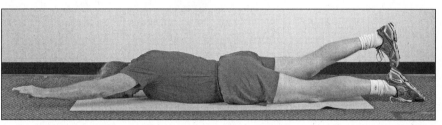

Photograph by Matt Bowen

If having your arms outstretched bothers your shoulders, tuck your elbows into your sides with your hands next to your shoulders. Instead of alternating your opposite arm and leg, lift both legs and both arms at the same time.

Swiss Ball Rollouts

This exercise combines the spinal stabilization of the plank exercises with the dynamic movement of the abdominal crunches (see the preceding sections). Swiss Ball Rollouts engage all the core muscles. All you need is a Swiss ball.

1. **Sit on your knees with a Swiss ball within arm's reach.**

   Sit very tall so your hips are in line with your spine. Place your fists side by side on top of the ball and straighten your arms with a slight bend.

2. **Tighten your abdominals while you roll the ball away from your body.**

   Roll until your elbows are resting on the ball and your hands are off the ball. See Figure 16-13.

3. **Exhale as you press down on the ball and slide back to your original position.**

   Lead with your hips as you return to the starting position. Your hips should remain in line with your spine without sagging.

4. **Repeat for the recommended repetitions.**

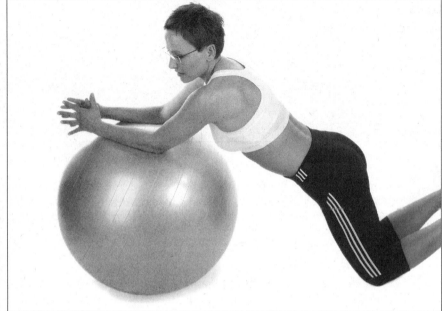

Figure 16-13:
Swiss Ball
Rollouts
engage all
your core
muscles at
once.

Photograph © Yuri/iStockphoto.com

Note: Because this exercise involves more movement than the planks do, it will probably make you sorer. You can make the ball exercise easier by using a larger ball or more difficult by using a smaller ball. Very advanced exercisers can graduate to an exercise wheel for maximum intensity.

Incorporating a stretching routine

Stretching your body parts is the third piece of the puzzle (the others being the basic weight training and core exercises we discuss earlier in the chapter). Most people tend to overlook this aspect of the workout because they feel it provides no benefit (which is flat-out wrong) or it simply hurts too much (which doesn't have to be true if you do it right). You don't have to devote hours to gaining flexibility. Adding yoga or Pilates to your schedule would be great, but just a few minutes of stretching each day can take you a long way.

Being flexible gives you the ability to compensate for accidental movements that may put you out of your normal range of motion without injuring yourself.

Here are some basic rules to follow:

✔ **Always stretch after you're warmed up.** The warm-up can include something as simple as stepping in place while pumping your arms. Stretching a cold muscle is asking for trouble. Think of your tendons and ligaments like a rubber band. A cold rubber band is very brittle and tends to break if pulled. Let it warm up a bit, however, and it becomes much more pliable and stretchy. That is how your connective tissue behaves.

✔ **Move into stretching positions slowly.** Never jerk or lurch into position. Hold the pose for about ten seconds, gradually trying to deepen the stretch. And don't bounce. Bouncing only triggers receptors on the tendons to contract the muscle. At the very least, you won't be able to stretch the muscle. At worst, you'll injure yourself in the process.

✔ **Focus on the area you're stretching.** Stretch right up to the edge of discomfort. You shouldn't feel any pain or tension anywhere except the muscle being stretched.

You can perform the following stretches in any particular order. We recommend doing them throughout your workout routine or at the end of the workout session. You can also stretch in between sets during your weightlifting workout, matching the muscle being strengthened with the muscle to stretch.

Calf Stretch

This stretch affects not only the calf but also the Achilles tendon in the lower leg and the plantar fascia in the foot.

1. **Stand facing a wall or chair back with both hands straight out in front of you against the wall or chair.**

2. **Bring your right foot forward, knee slightly bent; keeping your left heel flat on the ground, straighten your left leg as shown in Figure 16-14.**

3. **Move your hips forward while keeping your lower back flat.**

    Hold and then repeat with the legs switched.

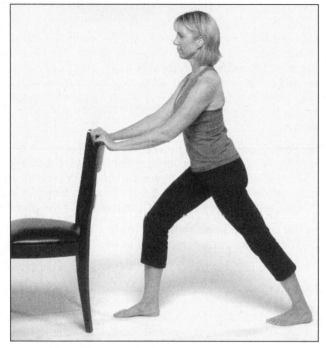

Photograph by Tilden Patterson Photography

Figure 16-14:
The Calf Stretch works the muscles in the lower leg and foot.

Quadriceps Stretch

This stretch affects two areas: the hip flexor and the quadriceps. Most people don't effectively stretch both of these regions. The hip flexor area becomes especially tight for most people because their lifestyles involve a lot of sitting.

1. **Stand tall and lift your left foot behind you, grabbing your left ankle with your left hand.**

   Support yourself by holding onto something with your right hand as shown in Figure 16-15a.

2. **Pull your heel toward your butt as shown in Figure 16-15b.**

   You'll feel the stretch in your thigh heading towards the knee.

3. **Pull your foot behind you away from your butt and stand very tall.**

   Your left knee should actually be pulled back slightly as well, causing your upper thigh to move backward. Now you should feel the stretch in your upper thigh near your hip.

4. **Repeat with the other leg.**

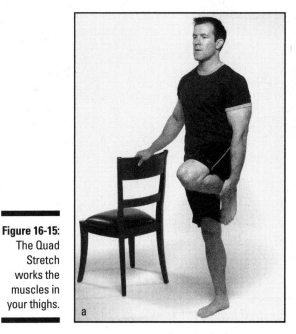
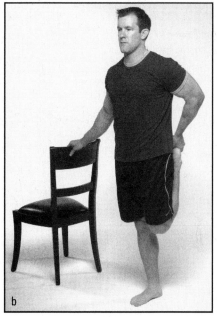

Figure 16-15:
The Quad
Stretch
works the
muscles in
your thighs.

a

b

Photographs by Tilden Patterson Photography

Hamstring Stretch

Tight *hamstrings* (the muscles in the back of the leg) are major contributors in the back problems that plague so many people. Without hamstring flexibility, folks tend to rely more on their lower backs when they bend over to pick up an object.

1. **Sit on the floor with your right leg extended; bend your left leg so the bottom of your foot is touching your right inner thigh as shown in Figure 16-16a.**

2. **Reach as far as you can toward your toes on your extended leg as shown in Figure 16-16b.**

   Don't worry if you can't touch your toes. Just focus on the stretch within your range.

3. **Repeat with the other leg.**

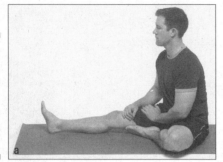
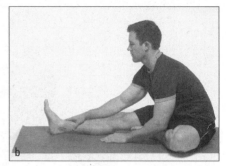

Photographs by Tilden Patterson Photography

Glute Stretch

Tight *glute* muscles (the muscles in your butt) are a common cause of knee and back pain. When glutes aren't functioning optimally, they can cause the surrounding muscles to work inefficiently. Thankfully, you can help avoid that with minimal effort and time.

1. **Lie on your back with your feet flat on the floor and your knees bent at 90 degrees.**

2. **Cross your left ankle over your right knee as shown in Figure 16-17a.**

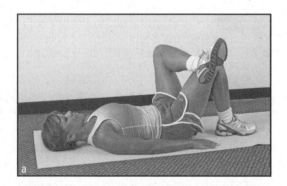

Figure 16-17:
The Glute
Stretch
stretches
the muscles
around your
hips and
butt.

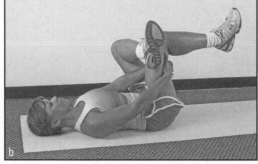

Photographs by Matt Bowen

3. **Reach with both arms extended and grab the back of your right thigh as shown in Figure 16-17b; pull your left leg into your chest.**

   Your left arm should be threaded between your thighs. You'll feel a deep stretch in your left butt and hip.

4. **Repeat with the other leg.**

Tricep Stretch

Unlike the standard tricep stretch, we recommend performing this exercise by tilting sideways and forward. This allows you to stretch additional muscle groups like the back.

1. **Reach your left arm overhead and down as if to scratch as low on your back as possible (see Figure 16-18a).**

2. **Grab your left elbow with your right hand as shown in Figure 16-18b and pull, allowing your left arm to reach farther down your back.**

   Tilt to your right and forward just a bit to also get a stretch in your entire left side.

3. **Repeat for the other arm.**

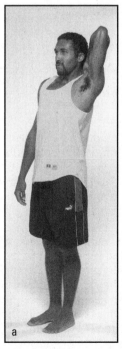 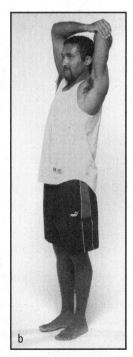

Figure 16-18: A modified Triceps Stretch works multiple muscle groups.

a   b

Photographs by Tilden Patterson Photography

Figuring Out the Details of Reps, Sets, Weight, and Rest

Determining the appropriate amount of resistance and numbers of sets and repetitions you should perform depends on your goals. These numbers will change over time as you progress and see how your body responds to varying these parameters.

Safety always comes first. If you can't perform an exercise with proper technique, lower the weight so you can execute the exercise correctly and protect yourself from injury. You can't speed the physiology of the body. It will adapt by getting stronger in its own time.

Taking a slow but steady approach to building up your fitness level

The stair-stepping approach allows you to start slowly and progress over time. This is the safest and most effective approach to weight training because you increase the number of repetitions and sets and the amount of weight in small increments.

With each upper body exercise, start with a weight that you can lift comfortably for one set of 15 repetitions for the first week of your training. During the second week, perform two sets of 15 reps with the same amount of weight as the previous week. During the third week of your training, do three sets of 15 reps and the same weight.

Don't increase the number of sets or repetitions or amount of weight if you miss workouts; your strength or endurance won't have increased as it should for you up the ante. For each workout that you miss, go back the same number of weeks and start your workouts at that level of sets, reps, and weight. For example, if you miss two workouts, go back two weeks and perform the workout you did then.

After you complete the first three weeks of your training, your body will begin to adapt to the training stimulus that you've given it and you can increase the weight. Increase the smallest amount possible, usually in 2½- to 5-pound increments. Reduce the number of reps to 10. When you can easily complete 10 reps, increase the reps to 12. When 12 becomes easy, increase the number of reps to 15. With each workout, continue with the same amount of weight until you can lift it 15 times with proper technique, and then increase the weight again. Continue with this stair-step approach by decreasing the reps back to 10 with each subsequent increase in weight.

With lower body exercises, start with an amount of weight that you can lift properly for one set of 20 reps. Increase the number of sets each week for three weeks as described for the upper body exercises.

During the fourth week of training, increase the amount of weight to the next weight increment. This amount is usually 5 to 10 pounds. Decrease the number of reps to 15 to allow your body to adjust to lifting a greater amount of weight. You can increase your reps with each workout until you hit 20 and then increase the weight again.

 Lifting less weight with more repetitions for lower body exercises ensures safety and prevents you from overloading your muscles. When you use more weight, your posture is often compromised because your leg muscles are so much stronger than your upper body muscles.

Matching your routine to your fitness goals

As a rule of thumb, the following repetition ranges lead to the adaptations provided. Consider your goals when deciding how heavy your weight should be. We also list a recommended rest period to help you recover between sets.

- ✔ Sets of 10 to 12 repetitions tend to build a mixture of *muscle hypertrophy* (an increase in your muscle size due to an increase in your muscle cell size), strength, and endurance. Rest periods of 30 to 90 seconds allow for the muscle to recover before performing the subsequent set.

- ✔ Sets of 15 to 20 repetitions increase *local muscular endurance* (your muscles' ability to repeatedly contract against a resistance over a period of time). Rest periods of 30 seconds are recommended in order to get the desired training effect.

These repetition ranges apply to most people; however, some people may find that they need to raise or lower the repetition ranges to get the desired results.

The number of sets you perform depends on your level of fitness and training experience (beginner, intermediate, or advanced). If you start at the advanced level before you're ready, you increase your risk of injury, excessive soreness, and overtraining. We list a sample workout week for each level in the next section.

Equally important to your workout is the amount of rest you take between sets. A 2.5- to 5-minute break between sets is best when your goal is to develop strength because it allows your muscles to recover at near maximum loads. A rest of 30 to 90 seconds induces muscle hypertrophy because you never fully recover but rather exhaust the muscle. When training for endurance, a 30-second rest works best because the resistance you're using is much less.

Designing Your Individualized Exercise Program

Want to create your own workout? Here are some pointers to keep in mind as you start:

- ✔ **Perform a five-to-ten-minute warm-up.** You can ride a stationary bike, walk around the block, or do a more functional warm-up such as hopping or skipping. You elevate your heart rate and body temperature and increase blood flow to the muscles you're about to start working.

- ✔ **Always stretch after having warmed up.** As we explain in the earlier section "Incorporating a stretching routine," you're more likely to injure yourself if you stretch a cold muscle.

- ✔ **Start with the largest muscle groups and move to the smallest.** For example, go from abs/lower back to legs, back, chest, shoulders, triceps, and biceps. (You can actually work your abdominals at the beginning or the end of the workout, but we recommend the beginning because it extends your warm-up without putting any stress on your joints.)

- ✔ **Never resistance train the same muscles on back-to-back days.** You need 48 to 72 hours to recover.

- ✔ **Your level of fitness plays a large part in what your volume of training should be.** Volume = Weight × Repetitions × Sets. (See the earlier section "Figuring Out the Details of Reps, Sets, Weight, and Rest" for more on these concepts.) For example, if you perform 2 sets of 15 repetitions with 10 pounds on the biceps curl, your volume is 10 × 15 × 2 = 300. The greater your fitness level, workout experience, and amount of resistance, the greater your volume of training.

The following sections provide some sample workouts at each level of experience to help you get started. You can read about the specific exercises from these workouts earlier in the chapter. Remember to include stretching throughout each workout after you're warmed up. We also include suggestions for fitness classes, such as yoga and Pilates, to add some variety to your program and to provide different training for your body.

Don't lift a weight that's too heavy for your fitness level because of the injury risk involved. Use a weight that you can lift for 15 to 20 repetitions. Your leg muscles are significantly stronger than your upper body muscles. As you increase the weight on your legs to reach 10 to 12 repetitions, your knees, hips, and back become considerably stressed, and injury can occur.

In the intermediate and advanced routines, we talk about super-sets and combo-sets. A *super-set* is a combination of two exercises of different muscle groups — usually opposing muscle groups — performed back-to-back without any rest. A *combo-set* is a combination of two exercises of the same muscle groups performed back-to-back without any rest.

Beginner sample week

When starting any resistance training program, always start off doing less than you're capable of doing. You're establishing a feel for each exercise. Creating good exercise technique habits at the beginning is critical to developing sound practices later on.

The sample workout in Table 16-1 is for a beginner interested in muscular endurance.

Table 16-1	Beginner's Sample Muscular Endurance Workout
Day/Activity	*Specific Exercises*
SUNDAY: OFF	
MONDAY: Level 1 Pilates class	
TUESDAY: Walk for 30 minutes	
WEDNESDAY: Resistance training	Pilates Modified Hundred Abdominal Exercise: 1 set of 30 reps
	Plank: 1 set of 30 seconds
	Back Extensions: 1 set of 20 reps
	Squats: 2 sets of 15 reps
	One-Arm Dumbbell Row: 2 sets of 15 reps
	Dumbbell Flat Press: 2 sets of 15 reps
	Bench Dips: 2 sets of 15 reps
	Dumbbell Curls: 2 sets of 15 reps
THURSDAY: Bicycle	A 5-minute warm-up and 20–30 minutes in your target heart rate zone
FRIDAY: Yoga class for 30–60 minutes	
SATURDAY: OFF	

Intermediate sample week

The sample week in Table 16-2 includes a resistance training program for an intermediate exerciser who is interested in getting stronger or bigger muscles.

Table 16-2	Intermediate Muscle-Building Workout
Day/Activity	*Specific Exercises*
SUNDAY: OFF	
MONDAY: Resistance training	Plank: 2 sets of 30 seconds
	Pilates One-Leg Teaser: 2 sets of 30 reps
	Back Extensions: 2 sets of 20 reps
	Lunges: 3 sets of 20 reps (body weight only)
	Squats: 3 sets of 15 reps
	One-Arm Dumbbell Row (super-set with Push-ups): 1 set of 12 reps, 1 set of 10 reps, 1 set of 8 reps
	Push-ups: 3 sets of 15–20 reps
	Bench Dips: 1 set of 12 reps, 1 set of 10 reps, 1 set of 8 reps
	Dumbbell Curls: 1 set of 12 reps, 1 set of 10 reps, 1 set of 8 reps
TUESDAY: Choose one: Yoga class for 60 minutes or swim for 20–30 minutes	
WEDNESDAY: Stationary bicycle for 45 minutes	
THURSDAY: Resistance training	Swiss Ball Rollouts: 1 set of 20 reps
	Side Plank: 1 set of 1 minute, each side
	Back Extensions: 2 sets of 20 reps
	Squats: 3 sets of 15 reps
	Lunges: 3 sets of 20 reps (body weight only)
	One-Arm Dumbbell Row: 1 set of 12 reps, 1 set of 10 reps, 1 set of 8 reps
	Dumbbell Flat Press: 1 set of 12 reps, 1 set of 10 reps, 1 set of 8 reps

Day/Activity	Specific Exercises
	Bench Dips (super-set with Dumbbell Curls): 1 set of 12 reps, 1 set of 10 reps, 1 set of 8 reps
	Dumbbell Curls: 1 set of 12 reps, 1 set of 10 reps, 1 set of 8 reps
FRIDAY: Choose one: Level 2 Pilates class or run for 20–30 minutes	
SATURDAY: OFF	

Advanced sample week

Table 16-3's schedule is an advanced workout for someone who wants to get stronger.

Table 16-3	Advanced Strength Training Workout
Day/Activity	Specific Exercises
SUNDAY: OFF	
MONDAY: Resistance Training	Pilates One-Leg Teaser: 2 sets of 30 reps
	Plank: 2 sets of 1–2 minutes, each side
	Pilates Modified Hundred Abdominal Exercise: 1 set of 100 reps
	Back Extensions: 2 sets of 20 reps
	Lunges (combo-set with Squats): 4 sets of 20 reps (body weight only)
	Squats: 4 sets of 15 reps
	One-Arm Dumbbell Row: 1 set of 12 reps, 1 set of 6 reps, 1 set of 5 reps, 2 sets of 4 reps
	Dumbbell Flat Press: 1 set of 12 reps, 1 set of 6 reps, 1 set of 5 reps, 2 sets of 4 reps
	Bench Dips (super-set with Dumbbell Curls): 1 set of 12 reps, 4 sets of 6 reps
	Dumbbell Curls: 1 set of 12 reps, 4 sets of 6 reps
	Elliptical cross-trainer for 30–45 minutes

(continued)

Table 16-3 *(continued)*

Day/Activity	Specific Exercises
TUESDAY: Yoga class for 90 minutes	
WEDNESDAY: Sprint training	
THURSDAY: Level 3 Pilates class	
FRIDAY: Resistance training	Swiss Ball Rollouts: 2 sets of 15 reps
	Side Plank: 2 sets of 1 minute, each side
	Pilates Modified Hundred Abdominal Exercise: 1 set of 100 reps
	Back Extensions: 2 sets of 20 reps
	Squats (combo-set with Lunges): 4 sets of 15 reps
	Lunges: 4 sets of 20 reps (body weight only)
	One-Arm Dumbbell Row (super-set with Dumbbell Flat Press): 1 set of 12 reps, 5 sets of 5 reps
	Dumbbell Flat Press: 1 set of 12 reps, 5 sets of 5 reps
	Bench Dips: 1 set of 12 reps, 4 sets of 6 reps
	Dumbbell Curls: 1 set of 12 reps, 4 sets of 6 reps
	Stationary bicycle for 30–45 minutes
SATURDAY: Run for 60 minutes	

Chapter 17

Evaluating Your Wheat-Free Lifestyle with Testing

In This Chapter

▶ Getting a better understanding of cholesterol

▶ Testing for health baselines

You've just left the doctor's office and now can't remember what the heck he told you. You recall something about needing to watch this number or that number and the possibility of needing a cholesterol-lowering statin drug in the future. "Come back next year for your checkup, and we'll see how you're doing," he said. All you have to show for your visit is a few pieces of paper with numbers that don't mean anything to you. All you can recognize is "high" or "low" next to some of the test results.

If this scenario sounds familiar, don't worry. You share the same feelings that most people have when they leave the doctor's office. That's why in this chapter, we explain what the basic numbers are for and what they mean. We show you which blood markers give you the best picture of your overall health. In addition, we discuss thyroid testing because it plays a huge role in the big picture of health and well-being.

The bottom line is that your wheat- or grain-free diet brings fantastic changes to the blood markers that matter most, slowing and perhaps even reversing the negative effects of your old diet. Positive changes from year to year are great motivators to keep doing what you're doing. Also, don't be surprised by the look on your doctor's face when he sees how good your test results are and finds out you've eliminated wheat/grains, added sugar, and vegetable oils from your diet!

Considering Cholesterol and Its Role in Heart Disease

For years, the world has looked at cholesterol as the enemy. But your body actually requires cholesterol to survive. Here is a partial list of what cholesterol does for you:

✔ Allows cells to communicate with each other

✔ Promotes strong mental acuity

✔ Produces all the steroid hormones, which regulate metabolism; energy production; brain, muscle, and bone formation; emotions; and reproduction

✔ Makes *bile,* which allows you to digest and absorb fats and *fat-soluble vitamins* (those that require fat to transport them through the blood stream)

✔ Supports the immune system

✔ Acts as an antioxidant

✔ Makes stress hormones

As you can see, cholesterol is a lot more important than previously thought. Almost every cell in your body produces cholesterol throughout your lifetime. Actually, as much as 85 percent of the measured cholesterol in the blood is produced by the body, while only 15 percent comes from the food you eat. And your body tightly regulates it by adjusting production based on how much cholesterol you're eating. Eat more cholesterol, and your body produces less, and vice versa. So much for the conventional wisdom that tells you not to eat certain foods because of the cholesterol content.

The movement to increase wheat/grain intake since the 1970s has also vilified fat and the cholesterol that those foods usually contain. For many years, the standard advice has been to avoid eggs, meat, poultry, and some fish along with butter because of the high fat/cholesterol in the food. Sure, eating more grains reduces the intake of cholesterol; however, the increase in the rate of heart disease has proven the high-carbohydrate/high-grain diet to be unsound and misguided.

If your doctor has put you on a low-cholesterol diet for medical reasons, we don't advocate going off that diet without first consulting him.

Introducing Western medicine's big four

Your annual physical will nearly always yield a basic *lipid panel,* a blood test measuring overall cholesterol, LDL (low density lipoproteins), HDL (high density lipoproteins), and triglycerides. We refer to these markers as the "big four," and the medical community gives them a lot of weight.

The panel is called a lipid panel and not a cholesterol panel for a reason. LDL and HDL aren't cholesterol at all; rather, they're vehicles that transport cholesterol around the body. You usually hear LDL described as "bad" cholesterol and HDL as "good" cholesterol. Think of LDL as the cars that transport the cholesterol from the liver to various parts of the body; spreading cholesterol to the rest of the body has earned LDL the bad cholesterol label, even though distributing cholesterol is a very important job, as we explain earlier in the chapter. HDL, on the other hand, are the cars that drive the cholesterol from around the body back to the liver, where it's excreted. Taking up the excess cholesterol has earned HDL the good cholesterol label.

The conventional wisdom that has designated "good" and "bad" cholesterol is a bit outdated. Cholesterol is cholesterol no matter what car it's riding in. In fact, HDL can sometimes transfer their cholesterol to LDL for distribution. And the plot thickens: Sometimes the LDL actually return cholesterol to the liver.

Triglycerides are fats made in the liver. Total cholesterol is a measurement of the total amount of cholesterol that the LDL and HDL are carrying.

The following sections examine the actual panel and the recommended ranges for each component.

The unit of measurement seen on lipid panels is written as mg/dl. This represents milligrams per deciliter, and it simply shows how many milligrams of a substance is present in a deciliter of fluid — in this case, blood.

Taking in total cholesterol numbers

Your total cholesterol number represents the amount of LDL and HDL in your body. Your goal is to have a low total cholesterol number.

Level	*Category*
Below 200 mg/dl	Ideal
200–239 mg/dl	Borderline high
240 mg/dl and above	High

According to the Framingham Heart Study in Massachusetts, 50 percent of all people hospitalized with heart attacks have normal cholesterol levels below 240, and 20 percent have cholesterol levels below 200. So an "ideal" total cholesterol level doesn't give you a free pass to ignore heart health. Peer-reviewed medical research hasn't proven that having low total cholesterol in and of itself reduces the risk of death in a population.

Looking at LDL numbers

Your LDL number represents the amount of cholesterol that is being moved from your liver throughout the rest of your body. You generally want a low number to come back from your blood test. (An easy way to remember the goal is that the first *L* in LDL stands for *low,* so you want a low number in your test results.)

Level	*Category*
Below 70 mg/dl	Ideal for people with high risk
Below 100 mg/dl	Ideal for people at risk
100–129 mg/dl	Near ideal
130–159 mg/dl	Borderline high
160–189 mg/dl	High
190 mg/dl and above	Very high

A large peer-reviewed study from the Get With the Guidelines database published in the *American Heart Journal* (2009) found the average LDL number for people hospitalized with heart disease was 105 (close to ideal). Almost half of the people studied had LDL numbers below 100. The analysis covered more than 136,000 hospital admissions.

The LDL measurement is for the weight of the cholesterol in the blood at a given time. If LDL are cars transporting cholesterol, the lipid panel actually measures the number of people in the cars, not the number of cars. Measuring LDL levels over time to monitor trends is a better way to analyze these lipids, as we explain in the later section "Pointing out logistical problems with the big four."

Highlighting HDL numbers

Your HDL number represents the amount of cholesterol that is being returned to your liver from the rest of your body. In this case, the higher the number, the better. (Just remember that the *H* in HDL correlates with *high.*)

Level	Category
Below 40 mg/dl (men)	Low
Below 50 mg/dl (women)	Low
40–49 mg/dl (men)	Borderline low
50–59 mg/dl (women)	Borderline low
60 mg/dl and above	Ideal

Smoking, not exercising, and eating lots of wheat and sugar lower your HDL levels, the opposite of what you want to happen.

Tracking triglyceride numbers

Your triglyceride number represents the amount of fat made by your liver as measured in your blood stream. You want this number to be low.

Level	Category
Below 150 mg/dl	Desirable
150–199 mg/dl	Borderline high
200–499 mg/dl	High
500 mg/dl and above	Very high

Triglycerides are solely a product of consuming a high-wheat/high-carbohydrate diet and alcohol. Wheat and grains cause excessive rises in triglyceride levels. However, when you consume fatty foods that contain triglycerides, the blood levels don't change much because the body stops producing triglycerides on its own.

Using lipid panel ratios as indicators for heart disease

The ratio of total cholesterol to HDL is a strong indicator of future heart disease. For example, if your total cholesterol is 240 and your HDL is 60, then your ratio is 4:1 (240/60 = 4). The ideal ratio is 5:1 or lower for men and 4.4:1 or lower for women.

An easy way to start lowering this ratio is by exercising and cutting the wheat/grains and replacing them with more good fats. Your total cholesterol will drop, and your HDL will rise. In fact, HDL tends to rise steadily for many years if you follow this diet.

The most important numbers taken from the basic lipid panel involve both triglycerides and HDL. The triglyceride-to-HDL ratio has continually given the greatest indicator of future heart disease in peer-reviewed research. For example, if your triglycerides are 120 and your HDL is 40, your ratio is 3:1. A good ratio to shoot for is below 2:1. Between 2:1 and 6:1 is the high range, and above 6:1 is the very dangerous range. Additionally, a ratio of 3:1 or higher is a strong indicator of insulin resistance.

Just like the total-cholesterol-to-HDL ratio, a lowfat diet that recommends a lot of whole wheat will make both these numbers go in the wrong direction. Those who have cut wheat and excess sugar from their diets find this ratio drops like a rock nearly 100 percent of the time. Sadly, because most of the focus by drug companies has been on lowering LDL, HDL and triglyceride numbers can get overlooked. Even if your triglyceride/HDL ratio is above 6:1, your doctor may only mention it if your LDLs are in a good range.

Understanding your LDL-P level and its importance

Although in preceding sections we treat LDL as one reading, it actually has two components: LDL-C (what we refer to in other sections) and LDL-P. The *C* in LDL-C represents *cholesterol.* This marker is the total amount of cholesterol being carried in the blood but doesn't indicate how it's being carried (whether it's all in one car or divided up among several cars, so to speak). LDL-P (the *P* is for *particles*) actually gives an exact measurement of how many cars there are.

LDL-P is perhaps the earliest warning sign of insulin resistance. It usually precedes increased blood glucose levels and increased insulin levels by several years.

Soon after the LDL particle gets into the artery wall, oxidative (damaging) forces occur that tell the body to send help to get the LDL out of there. Special cells are sent in (monocytes, macrophages, and mast cells, if you're curious) to investigate. If they find few LDL particles, all is well. Too many LDL particles means the special cells can remove some but not all of them. The body realizes it's losing the battle, and the damage expands deeper only to have the body cover up the LDL with smooth muscle cells. This process causes the artery to narrow.

In essence, it's a numbers game. The more LDL particles, the greater the chance they end up in the walls of the artery, causing inflammation and plaque.

Check out everything that can raise your LDL-P number:

✔ A diet high in wheat and grain, processed and refined carbohydrates, sugar, and high-omega-6 vegetable oils

✔ A sedentary lifestyle

✔ Chronic sleep deprivation

✔ Environmental toxins

✔ Poor gut health

✔ Poor thyroid function or low T3 levels (T3 is the most active form of thyroid hormone)

✔ Genetics

Probably the best test for LDL particle number is called the *nuclear magnetic resonance* (NMR) test. It uses a simple blood test that can be drawn at all major labs.

In addition to measuring the LDL particle number, the NMR test tells you whether your LDL particles and HDL particles are big and fluffy or small and sticky. The idea is that the big and fluffy particles have a much harder time sticking to the artery walls, while the small, sticky, dense particles can wedge themselves easily into the artery walls. Although these subtypes of the LDL particles provide more details for the big picture, research seems to show that they're still not as important as the total particle number. Although large, fluffy particles are better than small particles, high levels of large particles can lead to heart disease. Your wheat and grain intake makes LDL particles small and sticky, so when you're looking at the overall picture of your health and diet, this is one more strike against the conventional recommendations.

Even though the NMR test is the best current method available for testing particle number, the results can vary for the same reasons that regular blood lipid panels can vary (see the following section for more on the shortcomings of occasional medical testing). Taking one test can only give you a piece of the puzzle. Getting an average from several tests is the optimal way to gauge your risk.

Pointing out logistical problems with the big four

Earlier in the chapter, we stress the need to look at the big picture when evaluating lipid panel results. That's not only because the individual numbers aren't necessarily indicative of heart disease but also because they can vary quite dramatically.

The lipid panel doesn't actually measure the LDL number at all; rather, it estimates it with an equation using the total cholesterol, HDL, and triglyceride measurements. This point is important because it means LDL is dependent on the others that are directly measured. For instance, LDL will fall if HDL rises, and vice versa. Another problem is that if your triglycerides are under 100, your LDLs will be overestimated.

Your cholesterol levels change at different times of the day and from season to season. For example, total cholesterol levels generally go up in the winter and down in the summer. Just like you can't determine overall traffic patterns on the freeway by monitoring them only at one time of day, week, or year, you can't get a complete sense of your cholesterol situation based on one isolated lipid panel.

One of the reasons cholesterol levels fluctuate is that cholesterol provides healing in the body. When the body's stressed from, say, an infection or a medical treatment, it produces cholesterol and sends it to the area where the damage occurred. When the wound heals, the body removes the cholesterol from the blood because it's unneeded, and cholesterol levels go back down. That's why people with chronic infections or inflammation have chronically high levels of cholesterol.

So how big a fluctuation are we really talking about? Research has shown that the differences can be as high as 20 percent in either direction! For example, if your total cholesterol comes back at 220 one week, it may report at 264 or 176 the next week. That wide range makes it hard for the doctor to interpret the results; he doesn't have an average but rather a snapshot in time. With a 264 cholesterol reading, most doctors would be very concerned and probably recommend a drug to bring the number down, while a 176 would likely get you a pat on the back. These two drastically different scenarios, though they're extremes, help illustrate why a single reading isn't necessarily an accurate picture.

I, Alan, have a personal story with lipid panels. I was having two separate markers checked that required blood samples to be sent to different labs. The nurse drew two vials of blood, one right after the other, and sent each vial to a lab for analysis. As a courtesy, each lab also performed a basic lipid panel. Guess what? The numbers were completely different. My total cholesterol differed by 11 percent, my LDL differed by 14 percent, my HDL differed by 6 percent, and my triglycerides differed by a whopping 84 percent! To me, this was all the more reason not to trust one single test for diagnoses. A doctor may have decided to put me on statins based on the results from one lab or send me on my way with a "healthy as a horse stamp" based on the results from the other lab.

The reality is that most people don't go to the doctor to get a lipid panel taken very often. At most, it's probably once a year during an annual checkup; every few years is likely more common. Think of ongoing monitoring of your cholesterol numbers as getting a second opinion on the results from a single panel. After all, if you were diagnosed with cancer, you'd certainly get a second opinion; why not take the same approach to cholesterol and heart disease?

Talking to Your Doctor about Other Health Tests

We recommend a few other tests in addition to the NMR test (see the earlier section "Understanding your LDL-P level and its importance"). These tests indicate your risk factor for heart disease without telling you whether your arteries are clogged. Bring this list with you when you go see your doctor. Surprisingly, many doctors don't request them, perhaps because they're less familiar with tests that weren't around when they were in medical school.

All the tests listed are common tests but, at the same time, aren't necessarily routine tests. In fact, you may find they were included in your last physical, but you didn't realize it or understand their importance at the time. Your doctor probably won't think twice about ordering them. We simply want you to realize the importance these particular ones play in knowing the status of your overall health. Knowing these numbers will also allow you and your doctor to make informed decisions about your care moving forward. Your physician will probably appreciate the fact that you have taken an interest in your health care.

Your doctor is working for you, so don't be afraid to question what blood tests he's ordering. Taking control of your diet should be followed by taking control of your medical care. If your doctor refuses to accept your request or isn't aware of the tests, find a new doctor. You can easily find other doctors who understand the importance of turning over every stone.

Seeing what other blood tests are available

Here's a list of additional tests:

✔ **C-Reactive Protein (hs-CRP):** Inflammation of the arteries is a big risk factor for cardiovascular heart disease. High concentrations of C-reactive proteins (CRPs) in the blood are an indicator of inflammation in the body. Of course, inflammation is a normal response to many adverse events — including fever, injury, and infection — so you shouldn't have the test done while you know you're sick. However, long-term inflammation results from a steady dose of wheat/grains, sugar, and high omega-6 vegetable oils.

A result of less than 1 mg/L indicates low risk for cardiovascular disease; 1 to 2.9 mg/L indicates intermediate risk; and greater than 3 mg/L indicates a high risk.

✔ **Fibrinogen:** *Fibrinogen* is a protein that determines how sticky your blood is. You want your blood to be somewhat sticky (so it will clot), but too much stickiness is an indicator of cardiovascular disease. Fibrinogen should be considered in context with other blood markers. If your other markers are good, your fibrinogen is probably fine; however, if your other markers are bad, you have another reason to cut the inflammatory foods from your diet. Smokers; people with high blood pressure, body weight, and LDL-C; and women past menopause usually have higher levels of fibrinogen.

Normal levels are between 200 and 400 mg/dl. There really isn't a treatment for elevated levels.

✔ **Lp(a):** *Lp(a)* is LDL attached to a protein called apo(a). In a healthy person, Lp(a) repairs and restores damaged blood vessels. If your body needs too much repair, however, it can promote oxidized LDL in the artery wall.

A reading higher than 30 mg/dl is related to an increased risk for heart attack and stroke. No drug is available to fix high levels, and lifestyle doesn't really affect the number directly. Knowing you have a higher Lp(a) would hopefully inspire you to cut the wheat, excess sugar, and vegetable oils so you can be as healthy as you can.

✔ **Homocysteine:** This amino acid byproduct causes sticky platelets to form in blood vessels. Like fibrinogen, a minimum amount of about 5 umol/L is needed by the body, but levels above 10 start to show increased risk for atherosclerosis, heart attacks, stroke, and blood clots. Folic acid and vitamins B6 and B12, which are all in short supply in grains, can decrease your homocysteine levels. Shoot for between 7 and 9 umol/L. Many of the autoimmune diseases that are caused or made worse by eating grains require drugs that increase homocysteine levels. You then have a double whammy!

✔ **Hemoglobin A1C(HbA1C):** HbA1C reflects your average blood sugar level over the preceding three months. The three-month average is a much better picture of your blood glucose levels than a fasting blood glucose test because the levels change by the minute even after a nighttime of fasting; the wider-spanning test takes these fluctuations into account.

Less than 5.3 is ideal. Under 5.7 percent is good. A range of 5.7 to 6.4 percent indicates pre-diabetes, and over 6.5 percent is considered diabetic. A high level indicates that either you're not producing enough insulin or you're insulin resistant and your blood glucose isn't getting taken up from your bloodstream. Both situations are very dangerous. Even small increases in blood glucose can be an indication that you're heading in a dangerous direction on the diabetes spectrum. (Remember, diabetes doesn't occur overnight; keeping tabs on changes in your blood glucose over time can signal that it's coming.) Cutting wheat and sugar will help lower this number for the same reasons it lowers fasting glucose.

✔ **Iron (Serum Ferritin):** *Ferritin* is a protein that helps store iron in your body. A test for it tells you whether you're in the correct range for iron stores. Iron deficiency (anemia) can wreak as much havoc in the body as iron overload. In fact, iron overload can contribute to heart disease. Because iron is stored in the body, the only way to rid yourself of it is through menstruation or donating blood, so men and postmenopausal women should never take supplemental iron unless prescribed by a doctor.

Ideal levels are between 40 and 60 ng/ml.

Tests for the thyroid

Research has shown that underactive thyroid, also known as *subclinical hypothyroidism,* is a major heart disease risk, especially in older women. The most common form is called Hashimoto's disease. Many times, this condition shows no symptoms and doesn't affect the results of the basic thyroid test, the TSH. The problem affects an estimated 10 to 20 percent of women and accounts for 90 percent of all thyroid imbalances.

The gliadin protein in wheat has a similar structure to the thyroid tissue. When gliadin enters the blood stream because of a leaky gut, the body not only attacks it but also mistakenly attacks the thyroid tissue as well, resulting in a malfunctioning thyroid. Cutting the wheat helps heal leaky gut and prevent thyroid disease.

Explaining the thyroid is really a book of its own, so here we only touch on some signs of underactive thyroid and what tests to ask for if you have the symptoms. We can't overemphasize the thyroid's importance; the thyroid is related to every system in the body, especially metabolism, growth, and the ability to process calories.

Some of the signs of a failing thyroid include the following:

✔ A hoarse voice (unable to clear your throat or speak normally), neck swelling, or snoring

✔ Weight gain or trouble losing weight

✔ Depression, anxiety, or mood swings

- ✔ Hormonal imbalances, including irregular menstruation or infertility
- ✔ Muscle or joint pain
- ✔ Fatigue, even after adequate sleep
- ✔ Cold hands and feet or feeling cold when others aren't
- ✔ Dry or cracking skin, brittle nails and excessive hair loss
- ✔ Constipation
- ✔ Poor concentration or poor memory

If these symptoms look familiar, ask your doctor to order the basic thyroid test, the TSH, for you. Depending on those results, you may need more advanced testing. The thyroid requires tests to evaluate the big picture, much like testing for heart disease does. A cascade of events takes place in the thyroid, and each test measures a different spot on the assembly line. Just because the line is working at the beginning doesn't mean it's working farther down the line. We recommend also undergoing free T4 and free T3 tests and a Thyroid Peroxidase Antibodies (TPOAb) test.

Chapter 18

Adding Supplements to a Wheat-Free Diet

In This Chapter

▶ Discovering why supplementing may be a good idea

▶ Figuring out which supplements you need

*O*ne of the biggest dilemmas you may have when starting on your new wheat-free/grain-free lifestyle is whether to take a vitamin or supplement of some kind. Many people feel that if they're making healthy lifestyle changes, they should do everything they can to be as healthy as possible. Usually, they think that means taking extra vitamins, but more isn't always better.

In this chapter, we discuss which vitamins and minerals you should consider taking and why. We also explain why you need to buy them from a reputable source. *Note:* The advice in this chapter is for the average person's general health and well-being. If you're facing specific health issues, talk to your doctor about what supplements you may need.

Understanding the Basics of Supplementing

Replacing the grains, processed sugar, and vegetable oils in your diet with high-quality, nutrient-dense foods ups your vitamin content tremendously. Packaged food is so highly processed that manufacturers enrich many products to add back lost nutrients.

The amount of a particular vitamin in a given food isn't the only factor to consider. You should get as many of your nutrients as you can from real food. You can't continue to eat poorly and supplement your way to good health. Nature has naturally packaged foods in ways that let the human body more easily absorb their nutrients. Research has continually shown that isolating a nutrient and putting it in supplement form isn't the most effective system for the body to use.

Deciding whether to take supplements involves several issues aside from food choices. In the following sections, we explain why you may need to enhance your diet with supplements. We also offer advice on choosing a source.

Recognizing why you need additional nutrients

The U.S. Food and Drug Administration (FDA) sets a *Recommended Dietary Allowance* (RDA) for nutrients; this figure is the minimum amount of a particular nutrient needed daily to prevent deficiency diseases, such as scurvy, rickets, and night blindness. However, taking just the minimum amount of a nutrient may not optimize your health and well-being.

Having too much of a nutrient may not be wise, either. For best health, you and your doctor need to find the amount that works best in your system and balances with other nutrients.

Although you eliminate less-nutritious foods and eat more healthfully on a wheat-free diet, the food available to you may not be as rich in nutrients as it should be. Food may be less nutritious because

- ✔ Crops are raised in soil that has been depleted of nutrients.
- ✔ Plants are treated with pesticides and other chemicals.
- ✔ Crops have been genetically modified to the point that their nutritional content is lower.
- ✔ Animals are raised in unhealthy conditions, fed corn rather than grass, and given growth hormones and antibiotics to fix the associated problems of *their* poor diets. These toxins then pass to the people who eat meat or dairy products from these animals.

Supplements can help adjust for these shortcomings in food. However, you may need to add supplements to your diet for other reasons, including

- ✔ An increase in exposure to environmental toxins
- ✔ The overuse of antibiotics, birth control, and other medications that can harm the gut and liver
- ✔ Too much stress
- ✔ Not enough sleep
- ✔ Not enough exercise and too much sitting for prolonged periods of time

All these factors place great demands on your nutritional requirements and can lead to inflammation and chronic illnesses. Cutting wheat, added sugar, and vegetable oils are a great start to combatting these hurdles to good health, but you likely still need a few extra vitamins. We talk about the nutrients everyone needs later in the chapter.

In addition, you may need to take specific supplements for a limited time to fix a particular condition. In those situations, make sure to work with your doctor and get tested.

Purchasing quality supplements

You can buy vitamin and mineral supplements in any number of places, from big-box warehouses to grocery stores, drug stores, and online retailers. The price ranges for similar products vary tremendously, but be wary of associating the lowest price with the best deal.

The FDA has only limited manufacturing regulations on supplements compared to its rules for pharmaceutical drugs. Supplement quality is really a product of the manufacturer's integrity. In a market as lucrative as the supplements game, ethics can get left behind.

Supplement manufacturers can cut corners by working with poor-quality raw materials, not using the active form of a nutrient, and incorporating additives, colorings, and fillers. Consistent dosing from batch to batch can also be a problem, so you don't really know what you're getting with each pill. Cheap synthetic vitamins fill most of the bottles on your average grocery shelf. A handful of companies supply the synthetics that are then relabeled by many different manufacturers, resulting in the exact same product being sold as different brand names. Throw in the fact that the number of choices can make your head spin, and it's no wonder the average consumer gets lost.

It's not just the quality of the actual vitamins that are important. Check the inactive ingredients for any offending additions. Supplement companies often add grain-based fillers like wheat germ, corn sources, food glaze, food starch, MSG, maltodextrin, hydrolyzed vegetable protein, and textured plant protein. Other common questionable additives include magnesium stearate, titanium dioxide, and stearic acid.

Be sure to look for supplements that contain very few inactive ingredients. Oftentimes, the label will say, "No fillers and binders; free of artificial flavors and gluten."

Despite these obstacles, a little research can help you choose a reputable company. Choose manufacturers that

- Follow the FDA's Good Manufacturing Practices (GMP), which include hiring qualified employees and instituting quality control procedures. (Check out www.fda.gov/Food/GuidanceRegulation/CGMP/ ucm110858.htm#manuf for a more-complete GMP list.)

- Rely on third-party analysis to verify all active ingredients and contaminants.

- Create products that were established from basic science, went through clinical trials, and have a long history of use and safety.

- Produce products free from sugar; artificial coloring and flavoring; preservatives; and additives such as shellac, chlorine, gluten, yeast, and lactose.

- List an expiration date.

Just because a product is expensive doesn't mean it has met these guidelines. Do your research, check the manufacturer's website, or call the company directly and ask about its standards as they relate to the guidelines.

What Supplements Should I Be Taking?

Lots of people take a multivitamin as "insurance" for a poor diet, but nothing can replace a proper diet for health. Too often, multivitamins contain too many of the wrong vitamins and not enough of the needed ones. That's why the following sections look at the needed ones while ignoring a multivitamin as an option.

The other reason we don't think you need to take a multivitamin is that with a diet void of wheat, added sugar, and vegetable oils and regular meals of nutrient-dense foods like meats and vegetables, you get most of your nutritional needs from your food.

Although the supplement amounts we recommend are generally safe, consult with your doctor about any possible drug interactions with other medications you're taking.

Magnesium

Magnesium ranks as one of the most important compounds in the body for overall health. Studies have consistently shown that most Americans are deficient in this mineral. Bad food choices and depleted soil levels are the likely causes.

More than 300 enzymes rely on magnesium for use in protein synthesis, muscle and nerve function, blood glucose control, blood pressure regulation, energy production, and the synthesis of DNA and RNA. As impressive as all those functions sound, that's only a partial list.

Higher magnesium levels reduce blood pressure by relaxing all the muscles in the body, including the heart. Magnesium dilates the arteries, making it easier for blood to flow freely. Higher levels also allow your body to better control its blood glucose levels. This in turn lowers the risk for diabetes and the inevitable heart disease associated with it.

We recommend everyone supplement with 400 milligrams per day of the chelated form. (*Chelation* is the process of combining minerals with amino acids, which makes them easier for the body to absorb.) Magnesium glycinate or malate are better absorbed and have fewer side effects than magnesium oxide or sulfate. The glycinate form should be taken at night because it aids with sleep, while the malate form should be taken in the morning for its energy boosting qualities.

If you're having muscle cramps, skip the bananas and try increasing your intake of magnesium. People often associate muscle cramps with a lack of potassium, so they eat bananas in hopes of warding off the painful muscle contractions. A magnesium deficiency is often the real culprit.

Fish oil for omega-3 fatty acids

One of the leading causes of inflammation is an out-of-whack ratio of omega-6 to omega-3 fatty acids. Omega-6 fatty acids are considered to be inflammatory, while omega-3 fatty acids are generally considered to be anti-inflammatory. Because inflammation is associated with almost every disease in the body, balancing these factors is of utmost importance. A body free of inflammation tends to be a healthy body.

Omega-6 fatty acids need to be in close ratio to omega-3 fatty acids; the recommended ratio is 4:1 or less. Most people's ratios are far higher than that because of modern dietary choices. Vegetable oils may be lower in saturated fat than butter, for example, but they have a high ratio of omega-6 to omega-3. Corn oil and soybean oil, which can be found in almost every packaged food, are in the 100:1 range or more.

A good wheat-free diet can help bring down your omega-6 numbers, but you want to make sure you're getting enough omega-3s. Eating wild-caught oily fish (such as salmon) is the best way to get your omega-3s. But if you can't seem to work a couple of servings of fish into your diet each week, supplementing with fish oil is an option.

Fish oil supplements are excellent sources of EPA and DHA (two omega-3s important for bodily function, particularly in the brain). Though your body doesn't absorb their omega-3s as readily as it does those from the actual fish, they're much better sources than vegetable-acquired ones such as flaxseeds. Our recommendation is to get about 500 milligrams per day each of EPA and DHA. Remember, more isn't better. Fish oils, like all unsaturated oils, can cause oxidative damage to the body, which is unhealthy.

If you already eat fish a couple of times a week, you may consider taking the fish oil every other day only. If you don't eat fish at all, we definitely recommend a daily dose.

Cod liver oil for vitamins A, D, and K2

Cod liver oil strikes a nerve with older generations because they remember their parents making them take it when they were sick. Its benefits to the immune system still ring true today (not to mention its effects on decreasing inflammation and improving heart function, glucose tolerance, and vision). The big difference now is that the options for flavored oils make the taste much more palatable.

What's the difference between fish oil and cod liver oil? The physical difference is that cod liver oil is taken from the livers of the fish, while fish oil is taken from the flesh of oily fish.

Nutritionally, fish oil supplies higher levels of omega-3 fatty acids (see the "Fish oil for omega-3 fatty acids" section for details about why you need omega-3s). Cod liver oil supplies lower levels of omega-3s but is rich in fat-soluble vitamins A, D, and K2. When these vitamins are in balance, they prevent the ill effects caused by having too much of any one of them. Here's a look at each of these vitamins in detail:

- ✓ **Vitamin A:** Some of the many benefits of vitamin A include aiding the immune system, maintaining skin health, fighting cancer and slowing tumor growth, and helping fight diseases caused by viruses, among other things. Some research has shown that high levels of vitamin A can be potentially dangerous, but when balanced with vitamin D, the dangers all but disappear.

- ✓ **Vitamin D:** Cod liver oil contains a naturally occurring form of vitamin D, which is associated with protecting against heart attacks and some cancers, promoting strong bones, and aiding in a healthy immune system. You can get vitamin D from exposure to UV light and from foods such as fish, eggs, beef liver, and pork.

Food/supplement sources of vitamin D become more important for those who use sunscreen and/or live in northern latitudes (especially in the winter), plus those who are older (your ability to convert sun rays to vitamin D diminishes as you age). For these reasons, research suggests that as much as half the world's population is deficient in vitamin D. That leaves supplementation (such as through cod liver oil) as the only option for many. (For more information about the health benefits of vitamin D, pick up _Vitamin D For Dummies_ by Alan L. Rubin, MD [Wiley].)

✔ **Vitamin K2:** Although vitamin K2 was discovered at the same time as vitamin K, only recently have scientists realized that K2 has a completely different function. Whereas K is involved in blood clotting, K2 plays a role in directing where calcium is deposited, mainly away from the heart and arteries and into bones and teeth where it belongs. It's also important for skin, brain, and prostate health. Food sources include cheese, pastured egg yolks, grass-fed chicken liver, salami, chicken breast, grass-fed beef, and _natto_ (a traditional food product made from fermented soybeans). Because most people don't eat grass-fed meats or natto, supplementation from cod liver oil is a good idea.

Why supplement omega-3s when so many food sources exist?

You have little danger of being deficient in omega-6 fatty acids because they're in so many foods. "But wait," you say. "I see omega-3s everywhere, too! Why do I have to supplement those?"

The answer is that not all food sources of omega-3s are equally valuable. Vegetable sources like flax, seeds, and nuts contain alpha-linoleic acid (ALA), which converts to the omega-3s EPA and DHA. But the conversion rate is poor, so the amount of omega-3s your body is using from these foods is actually lower than what you may see listed as the amount "contained" in the food. That's why we don't recommend relying on plant sources for your fatty acid needs.

That brings us to fish. Eating six ounces of oily fish with high omega-3 levels like wild-caught salmon, mackerel, sardines, or herring two to three times a week is recommended. Doing so while also mindfully decreasing your omega-6 levels is probably sufficient for a healthy person.

Remember: Farm-raised salmon that has been fed corn instead of eating its natural diet in the wild yields very low levels of desirable fatty acids. That's why we prefer wild-caught salmon.

If you're worried about toxins that may be stored in fish tissues, steer away from larger fish and fish caught in certain parts of the world (such as China and Thailand) where known toxins are higher. Check out www.montereybayaquarium.org/cr/seafoodwatch.aspx for help finding fish options low in toxins.

We recommend the fermented type of cod liver oil. *Fermentation,* meaning the oil is processed using digestive enzymes rather than heat or chemicals, maximizes the availability of the nutrients without harming the product in the process. Use the recommended amount listed on the bottle; because cod liver oil is a real food and not a manmade supplement, the exact dosage of each vitamin is inexact from bottle to bottle, so we can't give you a specific guideline.

How often you take cod liver oil may depend on your age and where you live. For those living in colder climates, we suggest a daily dose. If UV exposure is a regular part of your day, you may consider taking cod liver oil daily in the winter and every other day in the summer.

Probiotics

A *probiotic* supplement helps beef up the good bacteria in your system. Humans are exposed to probiotics from the moment they pass through the birth canal. During birth, bacteria from the mother moves to the infant, whose gastrointestinal (GI) tract starts developing "good" bacteria — probiotics.

Your gut has between 500 and 1,000 different types of bacteria, good and bad. By far, your GI tract houses the majority of your immune system. Many ailments arise from bad gut bacteria or flora, making it even more important to nurture the healthy bacteria in your gut. Unfortunately, modern overuse of antibiotics makes doing so difficult. When you take an antibiotic for an infection, you kill off the bad bacteria, but the good bacteria go down with the ship as well. Besides antibiotics, stress, extremely sterile environments, and processed food can disrupt your gut flora.

Our recommendation is to use probiotics only on an as-needed basis, not daily. Those times include coming off a course of antibiotics, recovering from a chronic illness, or going through an extremely stressful life situation. Heat damages probiotic supplements, so keep them refrigerated. Look for a supplement that has multiple strains of lactobacillus and bifidobacterium, and follow the label for dosage amounts.

Yogurt is advertised for its probiotic abilities, but don't be fooled by the marketing. Modern-day yogurt isn't like traditional yogurt in its raw and unpasteurized state. Today's pasteurized yogurt is void of most of the beneficial bacteria because of the heat involved in processing.

Part V
The Part of Tens

Some foods aren't as healthy as you've been led to believe. For a list of ten supposedly healthy foods that aren't, head to www.dummies.com/extras/livingwheatfree.

In this part...

✔ Out of 14,702 reasons to go wheat/grain-free, find out the top ten healthy benefits of this lifestyle.

✔ Keep your fridge stocked with healthy, wheat- and grain-free foods — even dark chocolate!

✔ Get the lowdown on ten obstacles to a wheat/grain-free lifestyle so you can recognize and overcome them.

Chapter 19

Ten Benefits of Living Wheat-Free

In This Chapter

▶ Discovering the fountain of youth (and energy)

▶ Eliminating the risk for a host of diseases

"I've been eating wheat all my life and I've never had a problem" is a common statement we hear from many a wheat eater. And it's probably true, or so they think. But some wheat-related issues don't seem like issues until you resolve them; you may not realize you had a lack of energy until you don't have a lack of energy. Some conditions, such as diabetes and heart disease, have a host of other contributing factors, so wheat may not jump to the top of your list of suspects. And other issues arise that you and your doctor may not associate with diet, such as an autoimmune disease or a gastrointestinal (GI) disorder.

In this chapter, we present ten ways giving up wheat can prevent or slow various maladies. Many people claim these conditions are an inevitable part of aging, but those people have probably never seen what aging looks like on a wheat-free diet.

After you make the commitment to rid your life of wheat (and the sugar and vegetable oils that are often found in wheat products), you won't turn back. The occasional relapse to your old lifestyle and the subsequent ill effects will provide a quick reminder of your previous life, when you "never had a problem with wheat."

Ease Gastrointestinal (GI) Problems

GI complaints — such as gas, bloating, nausea, stomach pain, vomiting, and cramping — are by far the most common symptoms associated with wheat. Most folks don't associate these symptoms with this irritant because wheat is still commonly considered an important part of the diet. People usually call out something else, such as dairy or alcohol; though they may have issues with those items, more often than not they can trace the GI problem back to wheat when they learn of its destructive effects.

One easy way to find out whether wheat is contributing to your GI problems: Cut the wheat. Odds are you'll see improvement within days.

Turn Back the Clock to Younger-Looking Skin

The skin is a mirror of what's taking place inside the body. If your gut isn't healthy, your skin won't be, either. Gut irritation caused by wheat, sugar, and vegetable oil intake — and the inflammation that irritation causes throughout the body — directly affects the health of your skin. Here are just some of the ways wheat consumption can cause skin issues:

✔ According to the American Diabetes Association, 33 percent of people with diabetes have a related skin disorder. (For info on the link between wheat and diabetes, head to Chapter 2 and the later section "Lower the Threat of Diabetes.")

✔ An unhealthy lifestyle leads to impaired resistance from the skin after an infection or inflammation has occurred. Translation: Skin disorders are not only more likely to occur but also harder to control when they surface.

✔ Wheat raises your blood sugar; the resulting elevation in insulin levels is linked to an increase in pore-clogging sebum production.

✔ Wrinkles and lost elasticity are another product of longtime wheat consumption because of oxidative damage.

Reduce Your Risk for Autoimmune Diseases

Autoimmune diseases occur when the body mistakes its own proteins (called *self-proteins*) for external proteins and attacks the self-proteins. This response is actually appropriate because the body is doing what it was meant to do. Problems arise when the body is overwhelmed by resilient foreign invaders and the autoimmune system goes into overdrive. Autoimmune diseases are thought to occur because of a combination of environmental factors and specific hereditary components. For example, gluten is the environmental factor for people with the hereditary celiac disease gene.

The interesting thing about celiac sufferers is that they're much more likely to have other autoimmune diseases, such as rheumatoid arthritis, Sjogren's syndrome, and insulin-dependent diabetes mellitus. Wheat isn't a trigger for these conditions, but this link suggests that a breach in the gut wall leads to other autoimmune diseases

Protect Your Thyroid

The protein portion of gluten is called *gliadin,* which has a very similar molecular structure to the molecules of the thyroid gland. Some wheat-related gut issues allow gliadin to enter the bloodstream; when that happens, the body sends out antibodies to attack the inflammation. Unfortunately, the antibodies can't distinguish the gliadin from the thyroid, so the body goes after the latter as well.

Twelve percent of people in the United States develop thyroid conditions during their lifetimes. Studies show a link between gluten intolerance and autoimmune thyroid diseases such as Graves' and Hashimoto's. Researchers even go as far as to suggest gluten intolerance testing if you have one of these conditions.

Improve Your Weight Management

Cutting out wheat and sugar leads to fewer blood sugar elevations. Whole grains have been shown to increase blood sugar levels as much as a candy bar. When you have stable blood sugar levels, you have an easier time maintaining a desirable weight. Besides the inflammatory results of chronically elevated blood sugar levels (see Chapter 4), the body uses insulin to direct the glucose levels to where they need to go, including your fat cells. They don't call insulin the "fat storage hormone" for nothing.

Yes, your caloric intake will probably decrease on a wheat-free diet, which can also contribute to weight management. But unlike on diets dedicated to cutting calories, you don't notice the change because the nutrient-dense foods you're now eating provide a lot of satiety. (*Nutrient-dense* means the foods have a lot of nutrients packed into their calories.) That feeling of wanting more and more simply doesn't exist.

Prevent Hypoglycemia

When you have low, normalized blood sugar levels, you don't experience *hypoglycemia,* or low blood sugar, which can affect some people a couple of hours after consuming a lot of grains and sugar. (The preceding section has details on how grains affect blood sugar.)

The cure for hypoglycemia, according to most doctors, is to eat more wheat or sugar to bring blood sugar levels back up. The benefit from this reactionary response is only temporary and doesn't address the fundamental issue: ridding yourself of the excessive blood sugar drops. When you eliminate the glucose response from wheat, you don't have the roller-coaster effects anymore. Not only do the energy dips go away, but the need to eat several small meals a day also becomes unnecessary. Most people end up eating two or three meals at the most on a nutrient-dense wheat-free diet. You get an empowering feeling when you're not a slave to food to ward off headaches and mood swings. You eat when you're hungry, not when the clock says to.

Increase Your Energy Level

When people ditch wheat, sugar, and toxic vegetable oils, they notice an increase in energy. Whether the change occurs because hypoglycemia goes away (see the preceding section) or because the body relies more on fat for energy, you feel years younger. That daily need for an afternoon nap may disappear, or you may find yourself easing up on the coffee in the morning. Relying on your natural energy and not an artificial boost from caffeine is an amazing feeling!

During your transition to your new lifestyle, your body goes through a lot of adjustments. The body is amazingly resilient, but you may experience a few days of energy dips, dizziness, hunger, and brain fog. If these side effects happen to you, hang in there. Things get better soon.

Lower the Threat of Diabetes

Risk factors for Type 2 diabetes include being overweight and having high blood sugar and triglyceride levels, among other things. You can easily control these three factors with diet, and cutting wheat is the first step. We describe how going wheat-free affects blood sugar and weight in the earlier section "Improve Your Weight Management." Throw in the fact that excessive wheat consumption raises triglycerides, and you have the diabetes trifecta.

Diabetes develops over 10 to 15 years, so start combatting it now. Waiting until the doctor says you're diabetic isn't a good option.

Decrease Your Risk for Heart Disease

Your heart is an obvious benefactor from a wheat-free diet because when you reduce your diabetes risk, you also lower your chances of developing heart disease. (People don't actually die from diabetes. They die from the damage it causes to the heart.) Keeping blood sugar levels down and reducing inflammatory response prevents cholesterol from being deposited in the artery walls. No inflammation means no heart disease, regardless of what your cholesterol numbers may say.

Minimize Allergies and Asthma

Allergies and asthma are two conditions that are often ignored as symptoms of a gluten-related issue. A common misconception among many people, including doctors, is that gluten problems are black and white: you either have celiac disease or you don't. In reality, a large gray area of gluten intolerance and non-celiac gluten sensitivity (NCGS) exists that doesn't show up on a test for celiac disease. It does show up in your daily life in the form of symptoms, such as respiratory problems, that you've been attributing to other causes.

Cutting out the wheat can relieve both allergies and asthma. Wheat is a proinflammatory food; that inflammation leads to allergies and asthma. In addition, the steroids used to treat severe asthma increase insulin response just like wheat does. It's like adding fire to a fire.

Chapter 20

Ten Staples for Your Wheat-Free Diet

Most people are creatures of habit, eating from the same repertoire most of the time. Every household has its go-to foods, and in this chapter, we make sure yours fit the wheat-free lifestyle (which also means cutting down on other grains and sugar and eliminating vegetable oils). We've listed some nutrient powerhouses that will lead you down the road to better health and a better quality of life.

What you notice as you read through the list is the lack of processed food. Your new way of life probably won't involve anything in a box because even when manufacturers remove the wheat or splash claims of "gluten-free" on the label, they've usually replaced the wheat with other undesirable ingredients.

Our list includes an assortment of snack foods, basics for main dishes, and even a little dessert to satisfy your sweet tooth. In time, you'll discover your favorites and will be able to tweak this list a bit.

Pasture-Raised Eggs

Did you know that one egg yolk contains more than 90 percent of the recommended daily allowance (RDA) of 14 nutrients? It even includes 100 percent of the RDA for vitamins A, D, E, and K. This superfood practically replaces a vitamin pill. And don't forget protein. Most people think the egg white supplies all the egg's protein, but the yolk actually contains more than 40 percent of the protein content in an egg.

Pasture-raised eggs raise the bar even more. The eggs from pasture-raised chickens have twice the omega-3 fatty acid content, three times more vitamin E, and seven times more beta carotene than typical eggs. These are eggs from happy chickens who are allowed to roam free. A happy chicken is a healthy chicken — one that doesn't need antibiotics, antidepressants, or ibuprofen, three drugs commonly found in chicken breast analysis.

Don't be fooled by the misleading term *free-range*. It just means the chickens have access to the outdoors; it doesn't mean they take advantage of it.

Keep some hard-boiled pasture-raised eggs on hand in the fridge or whip some uncooked eggs up into an omelet with a dark leafy green, some cheese, and avocado. Good eatin' for any meal!

Grass-Fed Beef

Grass-fed beef is another superfood. You can't beat grass-fed beef for nutrient density. First, it has two to five times the omega-3 levels of grain-fed cows. Then factor in its higher levels of conjugated linoleic acid (an antioxidant), beta carotene, vitamin E, iron, phosphorus, zinc, and potassium. Unfortunately, grain-fed cows are more desirable for ranchers because they fatten up at a much faster rate (the cows, not the ranchers).

Grass-fed beef tends to be higher in protein and lower in fat than conventionally raised beef, so it requires about 30 percent less time to cook. It's best cooked at medium temperature and only to medium-rare at most. After you get a taste of the good stuff, you won't go back.

Grass-Fed Cheese

Everything tastes better with cheese. Even cheese tastes better with cheese. Cheese has calcium, good fat, and protein that doesn't raise blood sugar levels. At the same time, it's very satiating, so it curbs hunger.

Of course, we're talking about cheese from grass-fed animals, not the products that try and pass for cheese (such as American cheese, those processed loaf cheeses, or shredded cheeses that have very long ingredient lists). You can get grass-fed cheeses raw or pasteurized, although finding the raw variety can be difficult unless you venture to a health food store or know a local farmer. That's okay. The pasteurized version will do just fine. Even people sensitive to dairy usually do well with certain grass-fed cheeses because very little lactose remains after the aging process.

Grass-Fed Butter

Another nutrient-dense powerhouse that tastes so good you'd think it was bad for you: grass-fed butter. Grass-fed butter has a darker yellow color than its inferior grain-fed cousin because of its carotene and vitamin A content. It also has an equal balance of omega-6 to omega-3 fatty acids, which is extremely important for reducing inflammation.

We recommend grass-fed butter, but keep in mind that using even regular butter is better than using the highly toxic, high omega-6 vegetable oils.

Butter will burn at high temperatures, so cook with it at low temperatures.

Berries

When you've banished most other sugar from your life and your tastes have changed, fruit takes on a whole new flavor, tasting sweeter than you ever could've imagined.

Berries are the most desirable of all fruits because you can reap the benefits of their antioxidants without unduly raising your blood sugar levels. Of course, you should always consume the raw fruit and not a fruit juice version. The fiber content in the raw fruit helps keep blood sugar levels down by slowing the digestion process.

Whatever your berries of choice — blueberries, blackberries, raspberries, strawberries — you can enjoy them fresh as a side with any meal or frozen as a base for a smoothie. Just be sure to get the organic variety if possible because berries sprayed with pesticides tend to absorb those pesticides.

Dark Leafy Greens

Calorie for calorie, greens are one of the most nutrient-dense foods on earth. Take your pick from kale; spinach; watercress; Swiss chard; and collard, mustard, and turnip greens. They're full of vitamins, minerals, and phytochemicals that fight off disease. They're also a good fiber source.

Plan on trying to get some greens with every meal, whether you make them the base of a salad, throw them into an omelet with your pasture-raised eggs, or just sauté them with some coconut oil or grass-fed butter and garlic as a nice side dish. (We discuss pasture-raised eggs, coconut oil, and grass-fed butter elsewhere in this chapter.) *Note:* Because of their bitter taste, collard and turnip greens are best used for soups or in slow cooker recipes.

Coconut Oil

This oil is made up mostly of *medium-chain triglycerides,* a type of fat also found in mother's milk. It's great for cooking at higher heats because it's not susceptible to unhealthy oxidative damage like vegetable oils are. Coconut oil acts as an antioxidant, aids in cholesterol control, boosts thyroid function, and is great for hair and skin, among many other benefits.

The uses for this amazing food are almost endless. Besides sautéing, coconut oil is great to add to a smoothie to increase your fat levels and acts as a shot of energy. Also, use it in your coffee, or even on your skin as a moisturizer.

Dark Chocolate

Just the word chocolate jump-starts most people's salivary glands. Don't add the dark chocolate version of your favorite candy bar to your shopping list just yet, though. The chocolate we're talking about isn't the stuff sitting in the grocery store checkout lane. Those bars have all sorts of unhealthy ingredients — such as sugar in various forms, soy lecithin, emulsifiers, and artificial flavors — and not a high enough percentage of cacao to trigger its health benefits.

When we say "dark chocolate," we mean chocolate with a cacao content of at least 70 percent. As the cacao percentage goes up, most of the questionable ingredients disappear. You're left with a treat that's loaded with antioxidants and is good for your heart, brain, and blood sugar control. Because the lower sugar levels don't trigger a binge, you can satisfy a sweet tooth with just a small serving (up to 3 ounces).

If you're worried about your high-cacao chocolate tasting bitter, remember that when you cut down on your sugar intake, foods that didn't taste sweet before become sweeter. Dark chocolate is no different. The bitterness disappears, and the resulting taste is delicious. Your classic milk chocolate variety will soon taste like wax and chemicals. If you aren't used to the darker stuff, try starting with a bar in the 55 percent range and work your way up.

Nuts

The healthy fats in nuts provide a lot of satiety, so you don't feel the need to eat more and more. Nuts are an easy snack; they travel well, so they're great in a pinch when you're hungry and nothing else is available. Just be sure not to leave them in a hot car because they can become rancid. A couple of handfuls a week (a handful is about 1 to 2 ounces for most people) are enough to reap the benefits.

When buying nuts, choose the raw, unsalted variety or even the sprouted version, which makes them easier to digest. You can also soak nuts for a few hours and then rinse to allow the enzymes to break down, which is easier on your digestion. Toss your favorite nuts on a salad for crunch or eat them straight. You can also grind them to make homemade nut butters.

Almond Flour

We list this flour substitute as a staple, but with a caveat. Almond flour is good to keep on hand for those times when you want to splurge and bake up something yummy. However, almond flour is very dense (using many, many almonds to make a typical serving used for baking), so the omega-6 levels of these baked goods are too high to make them a regular part of your life. For the special treat, though, it performs admirably!

Chapter 21

Ten Things That Can Sabotage Your Wheat-Free Diet

. . . .

In This Chapter

▶ Recognizing internal roadblocks

▶ Looking out for negative external influences

. . . .

Stepping outside of your normal eating routine can pose challenges to your wheat-free diet. Any one or group of sabotaging factors can affect your wheat-free lifestyle, but by developing a plan specific to each obstacle you'll face, you increase your chances of success exponentially. Over time, these specific plans become established routines that create long-term stability and healthy dietary habits.

The pitfalls in this chapter are common to most people eating a wheat-free diet. We give you some tips to empower you to handle any challenge you face. However, no one knows you better than you. Developing your own set of techniques to better manage the challenges you encounter may have a greater success rate than simply accepting our advice to the letter. Do what works for you.

After you've committed to a wheat-free lifestyle and had success for a while, nothing can sabotage your way of life. You've formed new habits, and you don't even think twice about the difficulties of the following ten derailments. Life becomes life, and yours is wheat-free. You feel confident that you're making the choice to live this way. People around you can't help but notice your new energy levels and general sense of well-being. Sabotage isn't an issue. We promise you'll get there.

Poor Planning

If you don't have a plan and stick to it, you're setting yourself up for massive failure. Ignoring potential obstacles ill prepares you for the inevitable: You get stuck somewhere without a wheat-free option. Approaching your diet with a sense of commitment, accountability, and realism is what determines your success.

Within your plan, allow for obstacles to arise that challenge your determination. Developing strategies in response to each obstacle is the key ingredient of your plan. Answer the following questions; you can find guidance on each of these issues throughout this book:

- Where will you shop for your wheat-free food?
- What wheat-free recipes do you favor?
- Which restaurants will accommodate your wheat-free lifestyle?
- How will you address traveling wheat-free?
- How will you approach holidays and family celebrations? (Check out "Parties, Holidays, and Family Celebrations" later in this chapter for help on this question in particular.)
- How will you deal with eating at a friend's house?

Limited Understanding of Wheat's Harmful Effects

One sure way of sabotaging your wheat-free diet is to not fully recognize the harmful effects of wheat. If you don't approach the wheat-free lifestyle with a sound understanding of what wheat does to your body, you're more likely to quit and go back to your old ways or to some diet fad that comes your way. The more you know about wheat, the better. By staying up to date on the latest scientific information on wheat's consequences, the process of eliminating wheat long-term and making a lasting change becomes more and more realistic.

Stress

Cortisol, a hormone that increases during stressful times, has a way of enticing you to reach for that doughnut or croissant for comfort. But these calming feelings are only temporary. Learning to deal with your stress in other ways is essential to overcoming the urge to stress-eat foods laden with wheat.

Useful stress management techniques to help keep cortisol levels at bay include exercising, using breathing techniques, practicing mindfulness, meditating, and expressing gratitude.

The good news is that if you've eliminated wheat from your diet, you're less likely to indulge in unhealthy wheat-filled foods when the urge to feed your feelings hits. You're more prepared to make healthy choices in handling your stress.

Failure to Completely Eliminate Wheat from Your Diet

Cutting only some of the wheat from your diet is like dipping only your toe into the swimming pool; you don't get the full experience you would if you jumped in headlong. In the wheat-free scenario, that means you don't see the full benefits or reduction in symptoms. The most difficult challenge is that of overcoming your cravings. If you continue to eat wheat, you'll never kick the wheat craving.

The best solution is going cold turkey and eliminating all wheat from your diet. After your body adjusts to this change, it will thank you by losing weight, decreasing gastrointestinal distress, and reducing inflammation.

Lack of Self-Control

A lack of self-control where food is concerned leads most people to compulsively grab whatever food is at hand. Living for the moment only leads to greater frustration and less confidence that you can make a permanent dietary change.

Lack of self-control is usually a result of other sabotaging factors at play. Having a wheat-free plan in place, cultivating a wheat-free environment, understanding wheat's harmful effects, and reducing your stress strengthens your self-control.

Unrealistic Expectations

Nothing kills motivation like unrealistic expectations. When your expectations aren't met, you lose confidence in your ability to change your diet and in the wheat-free message itself. Understand that everybody progresses at an individual rate. Even though you may not be seeing the changes you want on the scale, know that your gut health, inflammation, and blood sugar are all improving. Living wheat-free isn't just about weight loss, anyway.

To avoid the trap of unrealistic expectations, know your limits. Chapter 5 shows you how to set tailored goals, called SMART goals, that clearly define your wheat-free lifestyle.

Environment

Triggers in your environment can cause even the strongest person to fail. Eliminating as many of these influences as possible not only increases your chances for success but also reduces the amount of temptation you experience. Consider these questions to determine whether you need to change your surroundings to create a successful atmosphere:

- Do the restaurants you go to accommodate your wheat-free lifestyle?
- Is your kitchen stocked for wheat-free success?
- Is the route you take to work or school free from wheat-filled restaurants that tempt you?
- Do you spend most of your time with people who fully support your wheat-free lifestyle?

If you answered "no" to any of these questions, think about whether your environment is really conducive to your wheat-free lifestyle.

Parties, Holidays, and Family Celebrations

When was the last time you went to a party, celebrated a holiday, or went to a family festivity that didn't have boatloads of wheat-filled foods available for consumption? The answer is probably never. Several tips to help you manage such events include

- Eating before or after the gathering
- Offering to host the gathering or bring your own wheat-free dishes
- Consciously thinking about what's most important to you (your wheat-free diet)

> ✔ Avoiding stressful situations and contentious relationships that may send you reaching for wheat-filled comfort foods
>
> ✔ Practicing self-control

A Spouse Who Isn't on the Same Page

Whether your spouse is out to actively sabotage your wheat-free efforts or is just not willing to make the same dietary commitment you are, having a honey who doesn't support your lifestyle can be a great challenge.

If your spouse is out to see you fail, you need to find out why and whether you can do anything to improve the situation. Or perhaps your spouse just lacks the self-confidence to change his or her diet or doesn't understand how harmful wheat is. Many folks think only overweight or out-of-shape people need a diet to ward off health conditions. Helping your spouse understand wheat's contribution to diseases such as Type 2 diabetes, heart disease, cancer, and Alzheimer's may go a long way in converting him or her. (Chapter 2 has info on how wheat consumption ties to various conditions.)

Do what you can to educate your spouse about your new lifestyle and help boost his or her self-confidence, but understand that your spouse may not be ready to make a change in this area right now. If that's the case, respect that choice while reiterating your need to be wheat-free.

Excessive Drinking

Excessive alcohol consumption can affect your wheat-free diet in several ways:

> ✔ Drinking alcohol has been shown to increase appetite.
>
> ✔ Imbibing in excess influences your decision-making process, which may lead you to make poor food choices.
>
> ✔ The consumption of alcohol often goes hand in hand with wheat-filled snacks, which wreak havoc on your wheat-free diet.

Keeping alcohol consumption to a minimum is the best approach. A 4-ounce glass of wine, 1½ ounces of hard liquor, or one 12-ounce gluten- or wheat-free beer is the maximum most people can handle without increasing their appetites.

Mixed drinks are loaded with insulin-raising sugar, so you should always avoid them.

Index

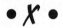

About the Authors

Rusty Gregory is the author of *SELF-CARE REFORM: How to Discover Your Own Path to Good Health*. He earned his bachelor's degree in physical education from Texas Tech University and his master's degree in kinesiology from the University of Michigan. He began his personal training business and became a Certified Strength and Conditioning Specialist with the National Strength and Conditioning Association. He opened Forte Personal Fitness, a personal training studio designed to help people become healthier through exercise, proper nutrition, and lifestyle change. He became a Certified Cancer Exercise Specialist with the Cancer Exercise Training Institute when he saw the particular needs that cancer patients have before, during, and after diagnosis and treatment. He is a Contributing Expert for dailyRx.com.

Rusty is also a Certified Wellness Coach. He helps people make lasting behavioral changes that lead them to become their best selves. Coaching has allowed him to become more empathetic with people and their wellness issues. He has seen many people realize a higher level of wellness and begin to live life with more depth, meaning, and purpose.

In writing this book, Rusty drew on more than 20 years of experience as a personal fitness trainer and wellness coach as well as his formal training and certification in both fields of study. His desire for continuing education has influenced the writing of this book and given him the tools to train people in a way that enhances their lives through health, fitness, and nutrition. To read Rusty's blog, visit www.rustygregory.com.

Alan Chasen has 25 years of experience as a personal trainer working in the field of strength and conditioning. Although he has trained people of varied interests, including sport-specific athletes, his true love is introducing the average person to a life of regular exercise, proper nutrition, and general well-being.

His journey started at the University of Texas, where he received his degree in Kinesiology at a time when personal training was still in its fledgling state. With a foundation built around physiology, anatomy, and nutrition, he has owned his own fitness studio since 1989 (visit chasenfitness.com for more information). Alan has spoken to many groups on various fitness topics, including the National Strength and Conditioning Association (NSCA) and the popular RunTex Austin speaker series. In addition, he consults on home and commercial gym designs.

This journey took a turn in 2009, when his dietary beliefs were challenged by what the science at hand made clear. The lowfat, high-carb philosophy that he learned from as early as 9 years old in Weight Watchers right through his college career was turned upside down when he realized that fat was good and carbs (including the so-called healthy whole grains) were bad. By relating his experiences and the science behind them to clients and others, he has been able to offer people the correct path to improved health and a superior quality of life — one that for most people cannot be achieved through a predominantly high-carb lifestyle.

Dedication

From Rusty: I dedicate this book to my wife, Karen, who understands healthy living. We have been on this wheat-free, low-carb journey together for several years, and as new research comes out, we learn and grow together. When I "checked out" of family responsibilities to write the book, she was always there to pick up the slack. I also dedicate this book to my children, Brittany, Lauren, and David, who supported and encouraged me throughout its creation. To my parents, Russell and Kay, who instilled in me the necessary work ethic to complete this project. To Dr. Andy Weary, who got the ball rolling and introduced me to the benefits of a wheat-free, low-carbohydrate diet, which turned my former way of thinking, upside-down.

I also dedicate this book to all the people who criticize and question me on the wheat-free, low-carb way of eating. They act as a source of motivation for me to learn and grow. Finally, to all my clients, whose friendships continue to support and push me to a higher level.

From Alan: I would first like to dedicate this book to my wife, Alissa, and my daughter, Sophie. They had to endure the sight of me sitting in front of the computer way too often while I was researching and writing. The recipes in this book are the usual fixings in our kitchen by Alissa. I am a lucky man.

I also want to dedicate this book to my parents, Hal and Celene. They have provided an emotional safety net throughout my life that can't be overlooked. Taking chances in life is always easy when your parents are your biggest fans. Dad taught me to "never settle," and Mom taught me that "everything always works out for the best." So far, so good.

Finally, I want to dedicate this book to my clients, also known as my extended family. Meeting with these folks two or three times a week for years and years has allowed me to have more intimate friendships than most people can ever imagine in a lifetime. I only hope I taught them as much as they've taught me.

Authors' Acknowledgments

From Rusty: Thank you to my business partner and coauthor, Alan Chasen, who I always knew was working tirelessly on his part of the book and was so supportive of all my writing as well. I am grateful for the invitation to participate in this project. I also appreciate Alissa Chasen and her help with the recipe chapters. Her knack for constructing wheat-free/low-carb recipes helped us provide delicious wheat-free food options.

I would also like to thank Rob Sterba, whom I've never met. His acceptance of this project and subsequent passing it on allowed me the opportunity to participate. Also, thank you to everyone at Wiley, especially Acquisitions Editor

Tracy Boggier, who gave me the opportunity to write this book, and Project Editor Vicki Adang, who was patient, informative, and very helpful throughout the writing process.

From Alan: A big thanks to my coauthor Rusty Gregory. His fear of the slippery slope kept us on schedule. I had to keep up with his determination. Working together was as easy as I thought it would be. Thanks to Rob Sterba. It never ceases to amaze me how people fall into your life seemingly for a reason. Without his trust in me and his introduction to Wiley, I would not have been an author.

I must also thank Dr. Andy Weary for changing the course of my life by recommending Gary Taubes's masterpiece *Good Calories, Bad Calories.* It took only 20 pages for me to experience as close to a spiritual awakening as I have had. It's crazy, but Taubes's book on nutrition and metabolism read like a murder mystery to me. Every page led me to question 30 years of education.

Thanks to my brother Larry, who received a call after those first 20 pages and answered the phone to "You're never going to believe what I just read." Your understanding and feedback as we have both learned the science over the last 5 years has been a comfort.

Finally, I'd like to thank the folks at Wiley, especially our editor Vicki Adang, for trusting Rusty and me with this opportunity. My passion for this topic is boundless, and I hope we exceeded your wildest expectations.

Publisher's Acknowledgments

Senior Acquisitions Editor: Tracy Boggier

Senior Project Editor: Victoria M. Adang

Copy Editor: Megan Knoll

Technical Editor: Nikki Jencen, CHC

Art Coordinator: Alicia B. South

Project Coordinator: Patrick Redmond

Illustrators: Kathryn Born; Elizabeth Kurtzman

Cover Image: © iStockphoto.com/Todd Harrison

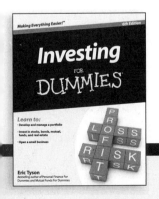
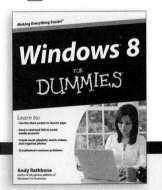
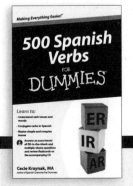
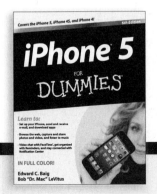

Math & Science

Algebra I For Dummies,
2nd Edition
978-0-470-55964-2

Anatomy and Physiology
For Dummies,
2nd Edition
978-0-470-92326-9

Astronomy For Dummies,
3rd Edition
978-1-118-37697-3

Biology For Dummies,
2nd Edition
978-0-470-59875-7

Chemistry For Dummies,
2nd Edition
978-1-1180-0730-3

Pro-Algebra Essentials
For Dummies
978-0-470-61838-7

Microsoft Office

Excel 2013 For Dummies
978-1-118-51012-4

Office 2013 All-in-One
For Dummies
978-1-118-51636-2

PowerPoint 2013
For Dummies
978-1-118-50253-2

Word 2013 For Dummies
978-1-118-49123-2

Music

Blues Harmonica
For Dummies
978-1-118-25269-7

Guitar For Dummies,
3rd Edition
978-1-118-11554-1

iPod & iTunes
For Dummies,
10th Edition
978-1-118-50864-0

Programming

Android Application
Development For
Dummies, 2nd Edition
978-1-118-38710-8

iOS 6 Application
Development For Dummies
978-1-118-50880-0

Java For Dummies,
5th Edition
978-0-470-37173-2

Religion & Inspiration

The Bible For Dummies
978-0-7645-5296-0

Buddhism For Dummies,
2nd Edition
978-1-118-02379-2

Catholicism For Dummies,
2nd Edition
978-1-118-07778-8

Self-Help & Relationships

Bipolar Disorder
For Dummies,
2nd Edition
978-1-118-33882-7

Meditation For Dummies,
3rd Edition
978-1-118-29144-3

Seniors

Computers For Seniors
For Dummies,
3rd Edition
978-1-118-11553-4

iPad For Seniors
For Dummies,
5th Edition
978-1-118-49708-1

Social Security
For Dummies
978-1-118-20573-0

Smartphones & Tablets

Android Phones
For Dummies
978-1-118-16952-0

Kindle Fire HD
For Dummies
978-1-118-42223-6

NOOK HD For Dummies,
Portable Edition
978-1-118-39498-4

Surface For Dummies
978-1-118-49634-3

Test Prep

ACT For Dummies,
5th Edition
978-1-118-01259-8

ASVAB For Dummies,
3rd Edition
978-0-470-63760-9

GRE For Dummies,
7th Edition
978-0-470-88921-3

Officer Candidate Tests,
For Dummies
978-0-470-59876-4

Physician's Assistant Ex
For Dummies
978-1-118-11556-5

Series 7 Exam
For Dummies
978-0-470-09932-2

Windows 8

Windows 8 For Dummies
978-1-118-13461-0

Windows 8 For Dummies
Book + DVD Bundle
978-1-118-27167-4

Windows 8 All-in-One
For Dummies
978-1-118-11920-4

Available in print and e-book formats.

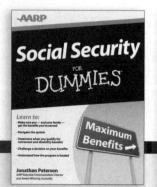

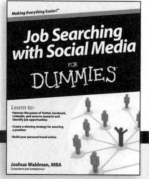

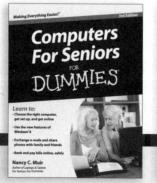

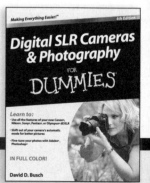